Path to Self Healing with Ayurveda & Yoga

Manual for mind, body and spiritual health
& well-being through one of the most ancient
healing methods.

ALYNA LIGHT

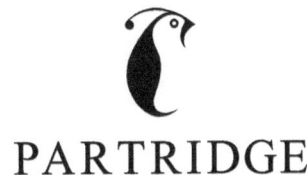

PARTRIDGE

To order additional copies of this book, contact
Toll Free +65 3165 7531 (Singapore)
Toll Free +60 3 3099 4412 (Malaysia)
orders.singapore@partridgepublishing.com

www.partridgepublishing.com/singapore

Contents

Acknowledgments

As I look back on my journey in search of natural and painless healing, it is clear that my experiences along this path have indeed been my greatest assets for acquiring valuable knowledge. What I have learnt and experienced are special gifts and blessings, and all these will not be possible without the help of special people I encountered along the way.

Here, I would like to express my sincere gratitude to my mentor (who prefers to be anonymous), for his guidance and imparting his great skills and vast knowledge with me during the course of my studies. I am always amazed by his enthusiasm and passion in teaching, his patience in healing people, and his continuous words of encouragement to boost confidence in others.

I would like to dedicate this book also to all my patients who have given me the opportunity to assist them in their healing journey toward better health. Their trust and support means a lot to me, and I am wholeheartedly grateful. Without them I would never have the chance to learn and gain experience and knowledge in integrative therapy.

Because of them, I have something beautiful to pursue, and it makes an important difference to my life and my personal growth.

Author: Alyna Light

Certified and qualified in ayurveda and yoga therapy and yoga wellness, and yoga instructor. Holder of diploma in holistic massage. Assisted patients with various health conditions such as osteo and rheumatoid arthritis, cancer, osteoporosis, diabetes, stroke, Parkinson's, kidney issues, digestive issues, menstrual, pregnancy issues, thyroid issues, asthma and sinus issues, back pain, shoulder and neck pain, knee pain, eye problem, ear problem, depression, stress and anxiety.

Introduction

Basis of Ayurveda Therapy

With an uninterrupted, unbroken tradition of more than 5,000 years, ayurveda is probably the oldest healing tradition known to humankind that has not only survived for such a long time but is still practiced in its original form. Its focus on self-care habits, conscious lifestyle, immunity, longevity, mental health, and holistic management of diseases have a universal appeal. The ayurvedic way of life seeks to enhance wellness through greater self-awareness, right diet and lifestyle habits, a union of body and mind (yoga), and the use of preventive herbs.

Healing in ayurveda is more about prevention and health promotion rather than remedial action. And when prevention fails, remedial action takes a holistic view of things, and not just focuses on curing the disease but also tries to prevent it from coming back.

Works on the Underlying Cause

Unlike mainstream medicine, healing in ayurveda is not all about treating symptoms. Its goal is to address the underlying cause of diseases early on. Ayurveda views all kinds of diseases as some form of dosha imbalance. Treating the symptoms of one disease may not help because aggravated dosha may again manifest as some other disorder in the near future. Therefore, unless the dosha imbalance is corrected, an individual is still at risk. Diseases are viewed as an effect, not a cause.

Ayurvedic medicines target this cause to prevent future occurrence of related diseases.

More than Medicines

Ayurvedic therapies do not solely rely on medicines. Along with medications, ayurvedic therapies include diet, yoga, lifestyle changes, as well as some preventive herbs to enhance immunity against similar kinds of diseases. Even after the course of medicine has ended, further lifestyle changes are suggested to sustain its benefits for the longer term.

Basis of Yoga Therapy

Stress is an outcome of today's lifestyle. It is produced out of wrong diet, fear, frustration, and dejection. At present, human existence is challenged by mental disorders or psychosomatic diseases such as dementia, hypertension, heart diseases, diabetes, asthma, etc. Although the ancient practice of yoga is not developed for the purpose of therapy, it has been observed through the continuous study that the regular practice of yoga not only controls these diseases but also prevents the developments of many diseases in our body. Though yoga is not an alternative therapy to modern medicine, it definitely supports the healing process.

Today, yoga practice is popular mostly because of its therapeutic value. Nowadays, the practitioner of yoga looks upon the care of his body as a primary duty. Yoga is undoubtedly the most effective and best suited to the demands of modern life. Yoga practice is a blessing for mankind, by means of its asanas, which give suppleness to the spine—our life axis, by stimulating and calming nerves, and by relaxing muscles.

Pranayama (the breathing regulation techniques) brings oxygen or prana to each and every cell and helps to burn waste products and expels the toxins from our body. Yoga has the potential to reduce stress and balance the mind, which is the key to the management of diseases. Therapeutic yoga is a holistic approach and works on the body, mind, and spirit simultaneously. The ancient techniques systematically strengthen each part of the body like the brain, heart, lungs, muscles, nerves, skin, and hair. Yoga also helps the body more efficiently to remove toxins or waste products, which are the main source of developing diseases.

The regular practice of yoga can bring physical and physiological changes. Hatha yoga says no two people are alike and have different strengths and weaknesses. So it's better to practice under the supervision of an expert therapist or guru to obtain the best out of it. Yoga is a slow medicine, but it is the best remedy for an uncountable number of diseases. Yoga therapy is a self-empowering process. The practitioner needs to adopt an incremental approach rather than aggressive strategies, which is more effective and key to success.

Chapter 1

How Ayurveda Therapy and Yoga Therapy Work Together and Contribute to Healing All the Five Layers of a Being

Ayurveda or ayurvedic medicine is the most ancient system of traditional medicine, which is native to India, that uses a various range of treatments, such as *panchakarma* ("five actions"), specified herbal diet and herbal medicine, to treat physical, mental, and spiritual health problems in order to bring health and well-being. Panchakarma is a fivefold detoxification treatment involving massage, herbal therapy, and other procedures.

According to ayurveda and yoga, our body is composed of five elements of *pancha bhootas* (pancha = five, bhoothas = elements). These five elements are agni (fire), vayu (air), akasha (ether), bhoomi (earth), and jala (water). These elements in different combinations characterize three types of doshas or bodily humors that make up one's constitution.

These three doshas are vata (air + ether), pitta (fire + water), and kapha (earth + water). These doshas become imbalanced due to diet, lifestyle, stress, etc. Whenever any of the five elements increases due to the change in dietary habits or lifestyle, it imbalances all doshas.

Hence, ayurveda therapy mainly focuses on the mind/body system and the balancing of the doshas. By changing or pacifying the imbalance of these doshas, ayurveda treats a person for both physical and mental

1

illnesses. Ayurveda in this way balances the physical, mental, and spiritual health of a person.

Yoga therapy on the other hand is mainly "shat kriyas" (six cleansings) or six detoxification procedures, which are essentially part of hatha yoga practice as described in the Upanishads (of Vedas). Shat kriyas consists of six groups of purification techniques. The main purpose of the practice is to balance the flow of two major nadi or pranic flows, ida and pingala, thereby attaining physical and mental purification and balance.

Other than the shat kriyas, one can use all other yoga practices like *yama* and *niyama* (the moral and ethical practices), yogasana, pranayama, and meditation for healing various types of physical, mental, and spiritual health issues.

The shat kriyas are classified as:

Trataka

Concentrated gazing for eye cleansing to purify the ocular system and also to cleanse the nadi system associated with the vision and brain. Also to activate the ajna chakra or third eye.

Neti

Neti or nasal cleansing using water (jala neti) and rubber catheter (sutra neti) for purifying the brain and nervous system and activating the ajna chakra or third eye.

Kapalabhati

Frontal brain cleansing using forceful exhalation techniques for lungs and frontal brain cleansing. Also, rejuvenates the digestive fire and digestive system and circulatory system.

Dhauti

Cleansing the stomach up to the intestinal tract. Vamana dhauti using water, vastra dhauti using cloth, and danda dhauti using rubber pipe. Dhauti of all types rejuvenate the digestive fire, energizes the digestive system, and cleanses the entire body and mind.

Nauli

Control of abdominal recti to cleanse the digestive system and rejuvenate the digestive fire. Purify the nadi system and brain.

Basti

Cleansing the lower gastrointestinal tract, especially the colon, removing toxins as well as cooling down the body.

Ayurveda therapy also uses the shat kriyas to balance the three doshas or components in the body such as kapha or mucus, pitta or bile, and vata or wind.

According to both ayurveda and yoga, an imbalance of the doshas will cause illness. Hence, shat kriyas of yoga therapy and panchakarma of ayurveda therapy is integrated to purify the body, and this practice will be used before pranayama (which is a higher yogic practice) to purify the body from the toxins for the successful progression along with the spiritual path.

According to yogic culture, our body has five layers or koshas, known as "pancha koshas." These are:

1. Annamaya kosha (food body or food sheath)

The material body or food body is made up of the five elements. Earth (prithvi), water (jala), fire (agni), air (vayu), and ether (akasha) are these five elements. The healing of any disease affected by this body can be done by both panchakarma of ayurveda therapy and shat kriyas of yoga therapy. Both panchakarma and shat kriyas are detoxification processes to eliminate negative energies and elements from the mind/body system. In a combination of both, one can purify not only the body but also the mind, and also the karmas of the past lives can be reduced or dissolved at a certain level. The integrative approach can balance all types of dosha imbalances and bring complete health to the body and mind.

Other than ayurveda and yoga therapy techniques, regular practice of yogasana, relaxation, and diet is also beneficial to bring well-being to the body and help them to achieve peace of mind and spiritual upliftment.

2. Pranamaya kosha (pranic body)

The vital sheath or pranic body is composed of five vital energies (pancha pranas) and five organs of action (karmendriyas) such as mouth, hands, feet, anus, and genitals. This body experiences hunger, thirst, heat, and cold.

Panchakarma and shat kriyas can rejuvenate and revitalize the energy channels for pranic flow and rejuvenate the body and mind.

Other than these therapies, the regular practice of pranayama can bring complete health to this layer.

3. Manomaya kosha (mental body)

The mental body constituted of (1) manas (mind), which is mainly thoughts and doubts; (2) chitta (subconscious), which is the storehouse of memories; and (3) jnana indriya (sense organs) for sight, sound, smell, taste, and touch. This body's work is thinking, doubting, anger, lust, exhilaration, depression, and delusion.

Panchakarma and shat kriyas can invoke calmness and restfulness to this body when the annamaya kosha is detoxified. Sattvic diet also can heal mental restlessness and agitation.

Meditation and chanting of mantras can bring healing of any mental illnesses and complete peace of mind and well-being.

4. Vijnanamaya kosha (intellectual body)

The intellectual body consists of (1) buddhi (intellect) for analysis and determining the true nature of any object and (2) ahamkara (ego), which is the self-assertive principle working with five organs of knowledge.

Decision and discrimination are its functions.

Shirodhara, a type of panchakarma therapy, is an important healing therapy for intellectual overdoing or excess analytical thinking. The brain can be healed this way. Shat kriyas such as kapala bhathi and trataka can bring calmness to the intellect.

Yoga recommends counseling, reading of classical texts such as Bhagavad Geetha, or philosophies like Patanjali yoga sutra, etc. can bring ultimate healing to this body.

5. Anandamaya kosha (blissful body)

It experiences bliss, joy, calmness, and peace. The main way to experience this body is by karma yoga in all circumstances, which give bliss in this body. It is the innermost layer and has limitless expansion as one experiences the bliss of life.

Chapter 2

Effects of Ayurveda and Yoga Therapy on Various Health Disorders

Ayurveda or ayurvedic medicine uses a variety of treatments such as panchakarma ("five actions"), specified herbal diet, and herbal medicine to treat physical, mental, and spiritual health problems to bring health and well-being. Panchakarma is a fivefold detoxification treatment involving massage, herbal therapy, and other procedures.

Ayurveda therapy mainly focuses on the balancing of the doshas. By changing or pacifying the imbalance of these doshas, ayurveda treats a person's physical, mental, and spiritual health.

Yoga therapy, on the other hand, mainly consists of "shat kriyas" (six cleansings) or six detoxification procedures, together with other yoga practices such as yoga asanas, pranayama, and meditation techniques. Shat kriya consists of six groups of purification techniques. The main aim of this practice is to balance the flow of two major nadi or pranic flows, ida and pingala, thereby attaining physical and mental purification and balance.

Let us see how ayurveda therapy and yoga therapy can be combined to heal various disorders .

Chapter 3

Healing Neurological Disorders

The term "neurological" comes from neurology and its Greek roots: neuro means "nerves," and logia means "study"—the branch of medicine that deals with problems affecting the nervous system. Neurological disorders are diseases that develop with the dysfunctions of the central and peripheral nervous systems. In other words, the brain, spinal cord, nerve roots, peripheral nervous system, resulting in physical and/or psychological abnormalities in the brain, spinal cord, or other nerves. Examples of symptoms include dementia, paralysis, sleeplessness, stroke, poor coordination, loss of sensation, and confusion.

Neurological conditions develop because of various causes, including genetic factors, traumatic injury, and infection. As per medical science, the causes of a few of these conditions are still not well understood. When we look at various neurological conditions, it can be grouped into four types:

- Acute symptoms – include headache, brain stroke, traumatic brain or spinal injury, meningitis
- Periodicals – include epilepsy, migraine, cerebral cavernous malformation
- Progressive – including Parkinson's disease, dementia, muscle weakness

- Stable with changing needs – include Tourette's syndrome, sleep paralysis, cataplexy

Researchers all over the world are actively investigating holistic therapies to find a solution to the global burden of dementia and other neurological conditions. According to the WHO data, around 50 million people worldwide suffer from some form of dementia, with about 10 million new cases reported every year. Humanity suffers from about six hundred kinds of neurological disorders. For most of them, therapeutic interventions of modern medicine have been very limited so far.

Therapy for Neurological Disorder

Every sick person suffering from the neurological disorder has a concern—whether or not it is possible to achieve full health again. Most of the time the answer to that question is "yes," and sometimes it's "no"; sometimes it's very difficult to answer. Apart from the issue of a restoration of full health, sometimes patients with neurological problems can be placed in rehabilitation centers as part of an effort to restore some of the basic functions. This is usually a bright and encouraging sign, as it's extremely difficult to find a patient assigned to therapy when there's dead hope for partial recovery. Therapy for neurological disorders may include:

- Change of lifestyle to either prevent or lower the impact of such conditions
- Regular physiotherapy practice to minimize the symptoms and restore some functions
- Headache, back pain, and joint pain management, as many impairments can be associated with considerable discomfort
- Timely medication under the supervision of a healer to either restore some functions or lowering the existing condition

There are more than six hundred known neurological disorders and conditions that affect the human nervous system, and for many of those, the treatment options are really limited because neurological disorders are the most complicated and complex disorders to heal as the nervous system functions are a basic, subtle, and complex system that coordinates all other systems in our body. Hence, the rejuvenation takes place slowly and with little or no response to the chemical-based treatment adopted by conventional modern therapy. This is the reason why ayurveda and yoga therapy can do wonders with these disorders. Both ayurveda therapy and yoga therapy can work in unison to make the rejuvenation and re-establishment of permanent health and well-being quicker and faster.

Ayurvedic Therapy

Ayurvedic therapies have a long history of remarkable success in treating many of these conditions. Since time immemorial, conditions like Alzheimer's, epilepsy, stroke, migraine, cerebral palsy, Parkinson's disease, and other degenerative disorders are being successfully treated with ayurveda. Various clinical investigations in the last two decades have also suggested the potential of ayurvedic herbs and self-care practices in preventing and reversing the progression of neurodegenerative diseases.

Vata Aggravation

Ayurveda defines neurological disorders as a condition of vata aggravation. Vata is one of the three bodily energies (doshas) that work in harmony with each other to govern all the physiological functions in the body. Vata, the energy of movement, is responsible for carrying out all kinds of transportations and communications in the body such as respiration, transfer of nutrients, working of the brain, neural communications, blood circulation, excretion, and working of the five senses.

When staying within bounds, vata provides clarity of mind, sharp senses, excellent cognitive capabilities, and creative thinking. However, when the body accumulates an excess of vata energy, it manifests as poor communication in the body. And since the brain relies so much on communication, it disrupts the working of our nervous system. In the short term, a person may experience brain fog, forgetfulness, difficulty in recalling a recently learned concept, or inability to think clearly. Over time, if the imbalance is not corrected for years, it may develop as degenerative neurological conditions.

Vata is characterized by light, dry, cool, rough, clear, moving, irregular, undisciplined, restless, and hyperactive qualities. Excess of any of these qualities, whether due to environmental factors, diet, or lifestyle, can increase its accumulation in the body. While individuals with vata-type constitution are more susceptible to neurological disorders, genetics and other factors may also play a role. However, in most cases, lack of awareness and ignorant lifestyle is believed to be the primary reason for vata aggravation. Balancing vata dosha and preventing its further aggravation is, therefore, the primary course of treatment suggested in the ayurvedic tradition.

The management of the treatment for neurological disorders can be divided into the following:

1. **Herbal preparations/herbo-mineral classical ayurvedic preparations**
2. **Panchakarma therapy**

Ayurveda considers neurological disorders as a result of a vata disorder. The vitiation of vata dosha causes an imbalance and disharmony in the human system that leads to neurological disorders. Ayurvedic treatments for neurological disorders will aim to rectify this vata imbalance and bring the vata dosha in harmony with pitta and kapha dosha so that it can eliminate the disease. Ayurvedic treatments include the use of ayurvedic medicines, panchakarma therapies like snehan (oleation/body massage), swedana (fomentation), virechana (medicated purgation), vasti (medicated enema), vamana (medicated emesis), shirovasti, shirodhara, padabhyanga (feet massage), murdha taila (head massage), and use of nadi swedana (herbal steam), etc.

Panchakarma is a series of holistic treatments that cleanse the body's deep tissues from toxins and open the subtle channels in the nervous system to bring life-enhancing energy, thereby increasing vitality, inner peace, and well-being.

Panchakarma is a fivefold treatment modality that is divided into three parts, namely purva karma (preparatory procedure), pradhan karma (main operative procedure), and pacchat karma (postoperative regimen). Panchakarma procedure purifies various systems of the human body and expels out the accumulated toxic metabolites from the body. Basically panchakarma is a bio-cleansing procedure that detoxifies the body and helps in increasing the bioavailability of drugs, diet, etc.

Purva karma (preparatory procedure): It includes carminative (deepan), digestive (pachan), oleation (snehan), and medicated sudation (swedan). These are beneficial for lubricating, liquefying toxic waste products/metabolites accumulated in various channels of the body and also helps for easy elimination from the body through the nearest route.

Pradhan karma (main operative procedure): After purva karma (preparatory procedure), as per requirement the pradhan karma (main operative procedure) like therapeutic emesis (vamana karma) and therapeutic purgation (virechana karma) has to be done so that one should follow medicated enema (vasti karma) and application of medicated nasal drops (nasya karma).

Pacchat karma (postoperative regimen): This is applied after every process of pradhan karma (main operative procedure). One should follow a special ayurvedic dietary regimen called samsarjana karma. It is important to restore the normalcy of body tissues and the system as well as rejuvenation of the person.

Some of the important oleation (snehan) process useful in neurological diseases treatment are:

- **Abhyanga** (body massage) together with **padabhyanga** (feet massage) for all neurological diseases except compressive neuropathy
- **Akshitarpan** for optic nerve atrophy, ptosis

- **Shirodhara** for insomnia, stress, cerebral atrophy, cerebral ataxia, Parkinsonism
- **Sirovasthi** for cerebral palsy, cerebral ataxia, Parkinsonism
- **Picchu dharan** for cranial neuropathy

Some effective sudation (swedana) therapy useful for neurological disease treatment are as follows:

- **Avagahan sweda** for all neurological disorders especially for neuropathy
- **Baspa sweda** for all obstructive uropathy

Herbs like brahmi are useful for the treatment of stress, insomnia, anxiety, depression, brain disorders, and psychosomatic and nerve disorders. Other herbs recommended include ashwagandha, bhringraj, and jatamansi. For centuries, these herbs are used to treat people to regain overall body strength and to alleviate many neurological disorders.

Brahmi

Brahmi is a premium ayurvedic herb for brain wellness, having been used to enhance memory and learning in children and adults alike for centuries. Brahmi is highly esteemed for its nootropic and neuroprotective abilities. It is traditionally used as a nervine tonic to strengthen the brain against various mental and neurological disorders like anxiety, depression, dementia, schizophrenia, and epilepsy.

Neuroprotective and memory-enhancing abilities of brahmi are well-researched and well understood. It is suggested as a potential treatment against seemingly irreversible neurological disorders, especially for Alzheimer's disease. One of the defining features of AD includes the presence of two types of abnormal structures in the brain: extracellular amyloid-beta plaques and intraneuronal tau proteins. Brahmi has been shown to inhibit the progression of both. According to a 2019 study, bacosides, bacon saponins, betulinic acid, and other bioactive compounds present in the herb exhibit significant neuroprotective abilities that protect the brain cells against oxidative stress, inflammation, and toxicity induced by plaques and tangles. A 2008 study also shows brahmi to possess powerful antioxidant abilities that can protect the brain against the harmful effects of oxidative stress and amyloid-beta-induced cell death.

A 2011 study has shown brahmi to prevent dopamine degeneration in old age, which may help in preventing and reversing Parkinson's disease. And unlike dopamine agonist drugs available for PD that become ineffective after prolonged use, brahmi remains effective even after years of continuous use. In fact, it is an herbal supplement ideally meant for long-term use.

Brahmi is profoundly relaxing for the central nervous system and is also a great sleep-enhancer. When taken during daytime, it can boost alertness and focus, while night-time intake pacifies the mind and induces sleep. Taking brahmi as a sleep-aid is not habit-forming and completely safe for prolonged use.

Recent research studies show that so many incurable neurological problems can be effectively treated by ayurvedic medicines, ayurvedic diet, and panchakarma therapies.

Ayurveda also recommends proper sleep because it is another great way to calm a restless vata energy. Loss of sleep, wandering mind, frequent dream interruption, poor sleep quality are symptoms of vata aggravation. In fact, sleep loss and vata disorders reinforce each other in a never-ending vicious cycle, which is why ayurveda recognizes sleep as one of the three pillars of health—along with diet and sexuality. Sleep is a natural way to detoxify and rejuvenate the brain. During sleep, our memories from the day get consolidated, important things are filtered out from the clutter, unnecessary information is removed, and the necessary ones are assimilated into the permanent memory. A good quality sleep of at least 7 to 8 hours, with enough time spent in the slow-wave phase (deep sleep), gives the brain sufficient time to perform these essential functions.

Sleep is also the time to reduce inflammation of brain cells, reset the brain's stress-response system, and remove amyloid-beta plaques. Amyloid-beta proteins are metabolic waste products that get accumulated in the brain and affect its functioning like memory, thinking abilities, cognition, and information processing. Accumulation of these toxins is the primary reason for developing neurological conditions like Alzheimer's and Parkinson's disease. According to the data available on the U.S. National Institute of Health website, sleep is essential for clearing out amyloid-beta proteins and can indeed reduce the risk of developing Alzheimer's disease. Several animal and human studies (1, 2, 3) have also linked enhanced sleep with reduced risk of neurological disorders.

Yoga Therapy for Neurological Disorders

Yoga is emerging as a widely practiced holistic science and integrative therapy. In a 2012 review paper that analyzed several studies conducted over the years, yoga therapies were found to be remarkably effective against many neurological conditions, including epilepsy, stroke, multiple sclerosis, fibromyalgia, and some disorders linked with the peripheral nervous system.

Yoga is a powerful source of treating many disorders and getting your health back on track. Yoga therapy for neurological disorders includes yoga breathing and warm exercises, yogasana, pranayama, and meditation. These practices should be done along with ayurvedic treatments.

Yoga breathing, warm-up exercises, and most of the yogasanas are good for the rejuvenation, coordination, and alignment of muscles and the nervous system in proper order and function, restoration of pranic flow in every cell and neurons and on the entire nervous system, balanced function of ida and pingala, which handles many of the neurological functions and balance of right and left brain functions.

Daily practice of thirteen rounds of surya namaskars followed by ten minutes' savasana or thirty minutes' yoga nidra can bring muscle and nervous system strength and coordination, high energy, emotional balance through left-brain strengthening, and mind-body balance.

Pranayama, especially nadi shuddi, ujjayi, and brahmari pranayamas, which are followed by meditation, are best for curing all brain and neurological disorders like insomnia, anxiety, depression, stress, cerebral palsy, cerebral ataxia, etc. and bring peace of mind and calmness to the body, mind, brain, and the nervous system.

Yoga is really amazing for the brain and nervous system. Its efficacy in various neurological disorders have been described below:

Yoga Nidra

Yoga Nidra is an important practice to control and manage neurological disorders. It is also known as "psychic sleep" or sleep in a state of inner awareness. A guided yoga nidra session helps to bring awareness to the sensation of heaviness throughout the body as well as to and from nerve impulses to the brain. After some time, however, the brain ignores these impulses and brings lightness to the body by improving the self-healing capacity. Regular session improves the feeling of lightness then the sick person restores health back on the track.

Asanas (Yoga Poses)

Yoga asanas are great to help to stimulate the nervous system and the spine. The nervous system is the network of ganglia that transmits nerve impulses or signals to each and every section of the body with the support of the spine. The following asanas are discovered and designed by our ancient yogis to control and cure neurological disorders:

- **Vrikshasana (tree pose)**

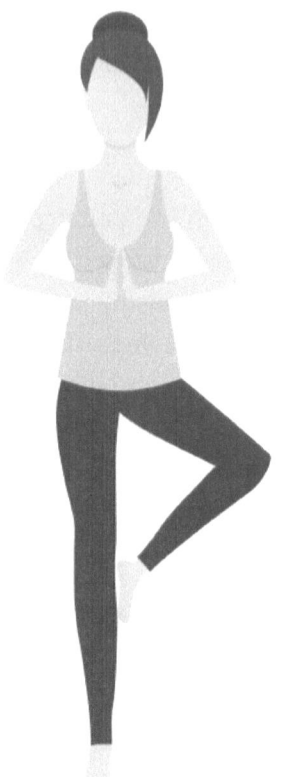

It strengthens the bones connecting to the lower limbs of the body due to the weight-bearing nature of the pose. This pose brings a state of rejuvenation. The one-pointed focus brings balance and equilibrium to your mind and helps to improve neuromuscular coordination, endurance, alertness, and concentration. A patient with neurological problems can practice this pose by taking the support of a wall or desk.

- Stand erect with legs hip-width apart.
- Using your right hand, bring your right foot up against the inner side of your left thigh.

- Find your balance, then place both palms together and as you inhale, slowly lift your arms up above your ahead or in front of your chest. Ensure that your biceps are close to your ears.
- Remain in this position and maintain normal slow breathing for five minutes.
- Bring your right foot down and repeat the same on the other side.

- **Balasana (child pose)**

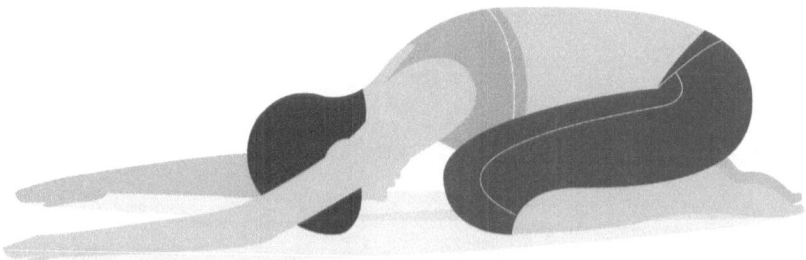

This asana is a great help to relieve fatigue. The person suffering from a mental disorder can practice it at any point in time. By stretching the spinal cord, it helps to reduce stress and anxiety. It stimulates the groin area, which helps to strengthen the circulation system vis-a-vis the nervous system by stimulating the core muscles and improving the digestion process. A patient with neurological problems can practice this asana for a peaceful sleep.

- Sit on your heels and keep your knees hip-width apart.
- Then slowly inhale and as you exhale, bring your chest down and rest it on your thighs.
- Stretch your arms forward in front of you.

- Relax and stay in this position while maintaining normal slow breathing for five minutes.
- Now bring both hands by the side of your knees, press your palms and slowly bring yourself up to the initial sitting position.

- **Halasana (plough pose)**

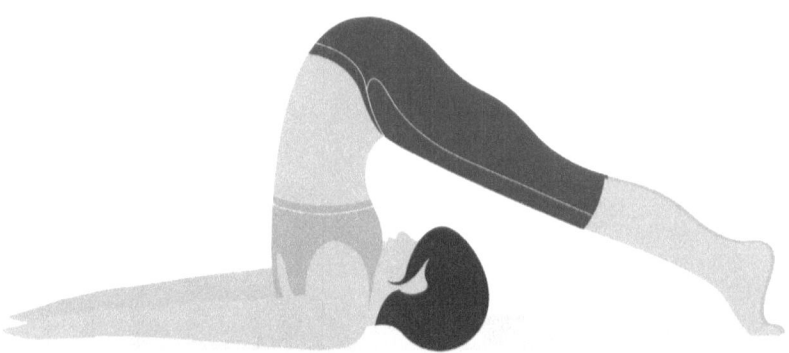

This is an advanced pose and looks difficult to practice but is really beneficial for the spine as well as the nervous system and its proper functioning. As it improves suppleness of the thyroid gland and the spine, in return it brings calmness to the brain and helps the speedy recovery of many neurological disorders.

- Lie down on your back, hands by the side of your body, palms facing downward and bring your feet together. Keep your body relaxed and take a few deep slow breaths.
- Inhale and slowly lift the legs off the ground using your abdominal muscles until they are at a 90-degree angle. Keep the legs straight and together.
- Support your hips with both hands and lift them off the ground.
- Bring your legs to a 180-degree angle over your head till your toes touch the ground. Your back should be perpendicular to the ground.

– Hold this pose for a minute while focusing on your breathing.
– After 1 minute, exhale and gently lower the spine and bring the legs in vertical position.
– Slowly lower the legs to the ground and let your whole body relax.
– Avoid jerky movements while releasing the pose.

- **Setu bandhasana (bridge pose)**

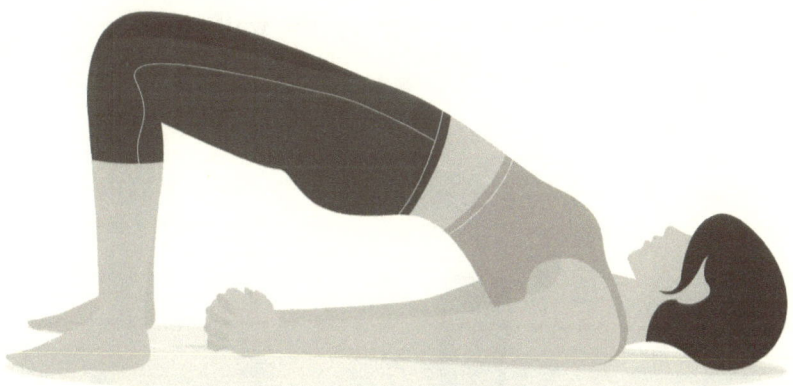

This beautiful-looking asana not only stretches the chest, neck, spine, and hips but also stimulates and strengthens the lungs, thyroid glands, and abdominal organs, the lower back, buttocks, and hamstrings. This asana is a great help to alleviate stress and mild depression and calms the brain and central nervous system.

– Lie down on your back, hands by the side of your body, palms facing downward. Your feet should be hip-width apart.
– Bend your knees and bring your feet close to your buttocks. Ensure that your ankles and knees are in one straight line.
– Press your feet and while you inhale, lift your spine off the ground, vertebrae by vertebrae.

- Now gently bend your shoulders and try to bring your chin to your chest.
- Let your shoulders, feet, and arms support your weight.
- Maintain this pose for thirty to sixty seconds with slow inhalation and exhalation.
- Then with deep exhalation, bring your back down and rest for a few seconds.
- Repeat the practice for three to five rounds.

- **Viparita karani asana (legs-up-the-wall pose)**

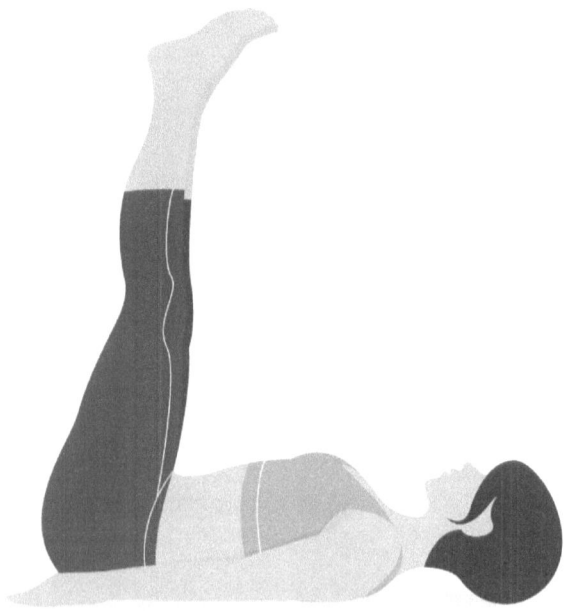

This advanced asana stimulates digestive organs and the neurons. This pose purges toxins out from the body and regulates blood flow thus helping to alleviate neurological disorders.

- Find an open space close to the wall and then sit right next to it in such a way that your feet lie on the ground spread in front of you. Ensure that the left side of your body is touching the wall.
- Exhale and lie down on your back, making sure that the back of the legs are pressed against the wall and the soles of your feet facing upward. You may need to move a little bit in order to settle down comfortably in this position.
- Place you buttocks slightly away from the wall or just press them against the wall.
- Make sure your back and head are resting on the floor. Your body will form a 90-degree angle.
- Lift your hips up and slide a prop under them. Alternatively, you can use your hands to support your hips and create a curve around the lower body.
- Maintain your head and neck in a neutral position. Soften and relax your throat and face.
- Gently close your eyes and continue with slow breathing. Hold on to this position for about five minutes.
- Release and roll your body to any one side. Breathe as you sit up.

- **Savasana (corpse pose) and relaxation**

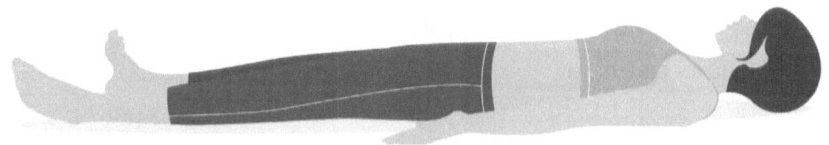

Always end the practice session with the corpse pose, as it is designed to relax and regain the energy. It reduces headaches, fatigue, and anxiety and calms the mind by reducing stress. A ten- to fifteen-minute practice of savasana calms the central nervous system and strengthens the immune systems.

- Lie down on your back. Feet apart, arms alongside your body, turn your palms upward facing toward the ceiling. Collapse your whole body, soften your facial muscles and make a beautiful smile.
- Close your eyes and inhale deeply and exhale slowly through the nostrils.
- Observe your whole body from your toes all the way up to your head.
- Now, at each inhalation and exhalation, relax your body part by part.
- Starting from your lower part (toes to hips). Sensitize the sole of your feet, loosen your ankle joints, relax your calf muscle, pull up your kneecap, relax the back and front of your thighs, relax your buttocks, loosen your hip joints and let it relax. Relax your pelvic region and your waist.
- Observe the changes in your lower part of your body for a few minutes.
- Shift your awareness to your abdominal region and observe the movements of your abdomen and chest rising as you inhale, and falling as you exhale. Relax your lower back, loosen your vertebral joints one by one, and relax your entire back and shoulder blades.
- Loosen and relax each of your fingers. Next, loosen your wrist joints and elbow joints and relax them.
- Relax your shoulders and relax your neck. The upper part of your body is completely relaxed.
- Observe the changes of your upper body for a few minutes.
- Lastly, relax each and every part of your head region. Your jaw, mouth, throat, nostrils, cheeks, your eyes, ears, forehead, side of your head, back of your head, and the crown of your head.
- Release your negative thoughts, tension, stress, and worry away at each exhalation.
- Stay in this relax position for about ten minutes.
- After ten minutes, bring back the awareness back to your body.

- Take a deep inhale, and as you exhale wiggle your fingers and toes.
- Then stretch your arms overhead to have a full body stretch from hands to toes.
- Bend your left knee, bring your right arm overhead and turn your body to the right side. Once you turn to the right side, your head will rest on your right bicep. Place your left hand on the floor in front of your chest. Press your left palm and slowly bring yourself up to a simple cross-legged sitting position.
- Take a deep inhale through your nostrils and slowly exhale through your mouth. Repeat breathing two times and then slowly open your eyes with a few blinks.

Pranayama

- ### Anuloma-viloma (alternate nostril breathing)

Regular practice of alternate nostril breathing comes as a blessing for the person suffering from a neurological disorder. The intake of fresh oxygen brings an abundance of prana to the body. As a result, the patient develops greater vitality, endurance, stamina, and strength. Moreover, the conscious control breath techniques develop neuromuscular coordination by increasing logical thinking and creative powers of the mind. Ten to twenty minutes of guided practice will bring positive signs to neurological problems.

- Sit in any comfortable meditative sitting position. Keep your spine straight, shoulders and neck relax.
- Adopt nasika mudra (bring your index and middle finger down).
- Close the right nostril with your right thumb and inhale through your left nostril. Make it as slowly as you can till your lungs are filled up.
- Now close your left nostril with your ring finger and release your thumb slowly and exhale through the right nostril.

- Next inhale through your right, then close your right nostril with your thumb and release your ring finger slowly and exhale through your left nostril.
- This is one round of anuloma-viloma (right and left side).
- Repeat another nine rounds.
- Once completed, you will feel that both nostrils are equally balanced, your whole body fresh and light.

- **Bhramari (humming-bee breathing)**

Bhramari is one of the best and easy pranayama to alleviate stress and cerebral tension by stimulating nerves connected to the brain. The regular practice of bhramari will strengthen the nervous system by stimulating the pineal and pituitary glands.

A patient needs to practice deep breathing techniques under expert guidance.

- Sit in any meditative sitting position. Keep your spine straight, shoulders and neck relaxed.
- Close your eyes and observe the sensations in the body and the calmness within.
- Now, close your ears with your thumbs. Put the index fingers above the eyebrows, and the other three fingers over the eyes.
- Take a deep inhale and as you exhale, gently press your thumbs on your ears while making a loud, continuous and rhythmic humming-bee sound (*mmmmm*) coming out from your throat.
- Feel the soothing vibration of the humming-bee sound over your face and other parts of your body. Continue this sound until the whole outbreath is out.
- Try to make a high-pitched sound for effective results.
- Repeat the same practice for three to five times.

Mindful Meditation and Relaxation

A number of studies showed unexpected benefits of meditation on neurological disorders. Benefits, from changes in brain volume to decreasing activity in parts of the brain involved with stress. Meditation is a form of mental training that aims to increase an individual's core psychological capacities such as attentional and emotional self-regulation. Guided meditation activates the parasympathetic nervous system and allows the patient to develop self-healing power for nervous system disorder, stroke, migraine, headache, dementia, Alzheimer's, epilepsy, etc.

Relaxation practices are considered the most effective treatments for vata imbalances. Excessive mental activity, lack of routine, anxiety, or chronic stress can further vitiate the restless quality of vata. Stress-reduction techniques like yoga and meditation have a grounding effect on the central nervous system and, therefore, can help keep vata in check. Ayurveda and yoga recommends mindful meditation for everyone regardless of body type or medical condition.

The benefits of mindful meditation are not unknown to the modern world either. Recent scientific developments in the field of neuroplasticity have opened a new vista of possibilities and changed the way we look at the capabilities of our brain. We now know that the brain constantly rewires, adapts, and keeps changing continuously according to experiences and environment. This is how meditation helps in healing. Mindful meditation is believed to have a positive effect on almost every aspect of well-being, including memory and cognition.

Various studies using brain-imaging techniques have shown mindful meditation to induce positive changes in the brain structure, such as thickening of the cerebral cortex, increased gray matter, and increased blood flow to areas linked with learning and emotion. In a 2011 study, an eight-week mindful meditation program increased the gray matter density in the hippocampus region of the brain, the region associated with memory, cognition, and information processing. The same study also reported decreased gray matter density in the amygdala, the region responsible for "fight or flight" stress response. These findings suggest meditation, especially mindful meditation, as a powerful tool to check the progression of neurodegenerative diseases. A 2018 study also recommended mindful meditation for patients of dementia, as well as for their caregivers.

Besides ayurveda and yoga therapy, another recommended therapy is cognitive therapy.

Cognitive Therapy

One of the primary and basic behavioral neurological issues goes by the name of cognitive-behavioral therapy (CBT), also known as talk therapy. CBT is a famous therapy that focuses on reorienting a patient's thinking pattern as well as behavior related to their disability, though it is not an appropriate remedy to many neurological disorders of the brain and nervous system.

According to a report from the New Jersey-based Center for Neurological and Neurodevelopmental Health (CNNH), CBT specifically administered in session format, where the patient is allowed free to engage himself/herself with the therapist in any way they wish, according to their present-day challenges, thoughts, and behaviors.

CBT is a collaborative therapy, requiring the individual and healer to work together. According to the American Psychological Association (APA), the person gradually learns various techniques to become their own therapist.

Naturopathic Therapy

- Since a healthy mind resides only in a healthy body, naturopathy advocates that the patient must live a natural life.
- The patient needs to get more sleep, even a few hours in the daytime, which will reduce tension gradually,
- Unpolished rice, milk, cucumber, mangoes, pears, guava, tomatoes, raisins, and leafy vegetables should be the mainstay.
- The patient should take periodical massage for reactivating the nervous system.

- The patient must be told to practice yoga, meditation, and other light exercises with his willpower to get rid of this disease.

Conclusions

Every person suffering from the neurological disorder is likely to make big changes to their lifestyles due to their physical inabilities, sense of perception, loss of memory, and reasoning.

They need to seek professional help as well as they need to follow above treatment methods, then it is very much possible to get rid of any nervous disorder.

Chapter 4

Healing Menstrual Disorders

What Is Menstruation?

Menstruation is a periodic change occurring in human beings and consists chiefly in a flow of blood from the cavity of the womb, and is associated with various slight constitutional disturbances. It begins between the ages of twelve and fifteen, though in warm climates and some races, it may begin earlier and in cold climates later. The duration of the menstrual period varies from three to six days and is a regular process in the majority of cases. The interval between the two periods is generally twenty-seven or thirty days.

Menstruation ceases between the ages of forty-five and fifty. The final stoppage is known as menopause or the grand climacteric. In the majority of healthy women, the normal menstrual cycle is of twenty-six to thirty days, with the exceptions connected with childbirth. Menstrual disorders are abnormal physical and/or emotional symptoms that arise before and during menstruation. Examples of such disorders are amenorrhoea (the absence of menstruation), menorrhagia (excessive bleeding during menses), and dysmenorrhoea (pain attending the process of menstruation).

The common menstrual disorders are premenstrual syndrome (PMS), irregular or absence of periods (amenorrhoea), painful menstruation (dysmenorrhoea), menstrual cramps, overbleeding (menorrhagia), etc.

Premenstrual syndrome is noticed with cramps, depression or mood swings, loss of focus, irritability, and craving for junk food. Polycystic ovarian disease (PCOD) also causes related menstruation disorders, like irregular periods and overbleeding, etc.

Amenorrhoea

Amenorrhea is a condition that arises because of the complete absence of menstrual periods for more than three monthly menstrual cycles. Amenorrhoea may be due to anemia, eating disorder, want of fresh air, excessive or strenuous exercise, obesity, and all causes, which depress the system and cause loss of flesh, tend to cause reduction and complete stoppage of the menses. Diseases like malaria, aggravated dyspepsia, and tuberculosis, as well as great grief may also produce scanty menses or totally stop them.

Dysmenorrhoea

Dysmenorrhoea may vary from mere discomfort to severe and frequent menstrual cramps and pain, accompanied by prostration and vomiting. Other possible causes may be because of pelvic inflammatory disease (PID), abnormal pregnancy, infection, tumors, or polyps in the pelvic cavity, smoking, consumption of excessive alcohol during their period, overweight and early menstruation (before the age of eleven). Sometimes anemia is a cause of painful menstruation as well as of stoppage of this function.

Menorrhagia

It is the most common type of abnormal/excessive uterine bleeding during menses and may be due to hormonal imbalance, pelvic inflammatory disease (PID), uterine fibroids, abnormal pregnancy, i.e., miscarriage, platelet disorders, high levels of prostaglandins (chemical substances used to control muscle contractions of the uterus), and kidney or thyroid disease.

Prevalent Medical Treatments

Discussion with the healer about menstrual disorder symptoms can help to determine the best treatment that will reduce or relieve your symptoms. Most of the time the trouble occurs due to lack of hormones. Hormonal imbalance is the main cause of menstrual disorders and PCOS. This happens because of stress due to overworking and overworrying, junk food, erratic lifestyle, and side effects of conventional modern medicines like antibiotics, painkillers, etc. According to medical science, the following therapies are available to control menstrual disorders:

- Diuretics
- Medicine through injection or taken in the form of tablets
- Vitamin supplements
- Dietary modifications
- Surgery for elimination of the uterus to avoid complications from excess bleeding

Ayurvedic Therapy

What a woman goes through during her menstruation could provide a useful insight into her physical and mental health, according to some gynecologists. More than 90 percent of women worldwide suffer from some form of menstrual disorder. In ayurveda, diseases happen when doshas go corrupt. Menstrual problems are also seen as a result of dosha aggravation. Different doshas are responsible for different kinds of menstrual disorders, and therefore the course of treatment also depends on the dosha responsible.

Weather changes, diet, nutritional deficiency, body-mind type, and wrong lifestyle are some of the factors responsible for aggravating the three doshas. A deeper understanding of self, right lifestyle adaptations, and personalized self-care practices can help restore the balance and provide a long-term solution to many of these conditions.

Vata Imbalance

Vata is responsible for all kinds of transportation in the body, including menstrual blood flow. When vata goes out of balance, it may lead to contraction of blood vessels and uterine muscles, producing abdominal cramps and pain in the lower back, shoulders, thighs, and legs. Psychological symptoms include stress, anxiety, mood swings, restlessness, and disturbed sleep. Individuals of the vata constitution may also experience missing or irregular periods because of the inherent irregular quality of vata. Autumn and winter seasons, overreliance on refrigerated food, indiscipline, insufficient hydration, lack of sleep, dry environmental conditions, and nutritional deficiencies are some of the factors known to aggravate vata. Here are some of the lifestyle changes that can help with vata-induced menstrual problems.

Nutrient-Dense Foods

Consume lots of foods rich in omega-3 fatty acids, such as salmon, flax seeds, olive oil, ghee (clarified butter), walnuts, and soybeans. Also, avoid light foods and go for nourishing whole grains. Foods rich in fiber, iron, magnesium, potassium, and vitamin D are also known to ease menstrual cramps. As a rule of thumb, try to balance the light, dry, rough qualities of vata with heavy, oily, dense, and smooth qualities of food.

Fresh and Warm Foods

Vata is cool and light. Ayurveda recommends eating freshly prepared meals for everyone, as refrigerated foods can further increase an already excess vata. Also, always warm your veggies before eating. Fresh fruits and raw vegetables (including salads) are not recommended for vata disorders. Instead, try steamed vegetables with yogurt or ghee.

Rest

Try to avoid rigorous physical and mental activities at this time, as restlessness negatively affects vata disorders. Taking a midday nap during cycles is considered very beneficial for relaxing the blood vessels and can help with mood swings and cramping.

Sweet-Sour-Salty

Foods with sweet, sour, or salty tastes help balance vata, while astringent, bitter, and pungent foods increase it.

Breathing Exercises

Simple breathing exercises are very effective against any kind of vata disorder.

Pitta Imbalance

Pitta imbalances are responsible for heavy bleeding, severe pain, irritability, anger, nausea, swollen breasts, and diarrhea symptoms. Sometimes, mild fever may also accompany heavy periods. Pitta aggravation also causes sharp hormonal changes in the body, resulting in irregular periods, acne, and mood swings. It may also trigger migraines just before or during periods.

Pitta is characterized by hot, sharp, penetrating, oily, smelly qualities. It can be balanced by opposite qualities of light, cool, dry conditions. Summer season, oily and spicy foods, stress, overly focused mind, and lack of sleep can aggravate pitta dosha.

Sweet-Astringent-Bitter

Choose sweet, astringent, and bitter foods over salty, sour, and pungent tastes. Turmeric, basil, bitter gourd, legumes, broccoli, turnip, coconut, and raw fruits and vegetables are great for calming pitta.

Unsweetened tea, coffee, coconut water, and fruit juices may also help in heavy periods.

Cooling Herbs

Herbs like amla (Indian gooseberry) and neem are excellent for pacifying pitta and help in the natural blood detoxification process. Amla is an incredibly rich source of iron and vitamin C, which helps replenish the body of lost iron. Iron deficiency due to heavy blood loss during menstruation can cause weakness, headaches, dizziness, and anemia. Amla is also known to ease blood flow and cramps.

Relaxation

Pitta imbalance is characterized by an overly focused and critical mind. Relaxation practices like meditation, music, sleep, and reading can help calm this quality. Some harmonizing essential oils like rose, ylang-ylang, lavender, clary sage, and roman chamomile oils are also considered beneficial for calming irritability, pain, and other PMS symptoms.

Kapha Imbalance

The heavy, dense qualities of kapha are manifested as bloating during menstruation. Some people also feel heaviness around the waist and thighs area. Psychological symptoms include heavy-heartedness, oversleepiness, and sluggish mind. Unreasonable hunger is also a kapha symptom. Warm, light, moving, stimulating qualities can help calm kapha-induced menstrual problems.

Avoid Emotional Eating

High intake of processed sugars, carbs, and salty snacks can worsen menstrual cramps. Instead, consider foods rich in micronutrients like vitamin B6, calcium, magnesium, potassium, and iron. Bananas are considered a wonderful remedy for bloating and can also help curb unnecessary eating.

Astringent, Bitter, Pungent

Choose light, astringent, bitter, and pungent foods over heavy, sweet, salty, and sour ones. Ginger, black pepper, turmeric, basil, clove, cardamom, garlic are some of the kapha-balancing foods.

According to ayurveda, a woman's body is in synchronization with the moon. That is the reason the twenty-eight days of the moon's cycle is in synchronization with the women's menstruation cycle. So any problems with the menstruation processes can be rectified with conscious living with the natural cycles of the moon and being with nature.

That is why the holistic medicines and treatments of ayurveda and daily practice of yoga become the best solution for all menstruation problems and also for PCOS. Hence drinking water every morning charged with moonlight on previous nights can help a lot to balance a woman's body cycles with the moon.

Also daily consumption of pineapples or pineapple juice can reduce menstruation complications as pineapple contains bromelain, an enzyme that softens the uterus linings and normalizes periods. Consume fresh vegetables and fruits for your meals as half of the portion, and add warm ghee to the food daily.

Ayurvedic Remedies for Menstrual Disorders

Ayurveda is pure sciences, which looks at the reproductive tissues outside of the major problems related to puberty, pregnancy, and menopause. Though ayurveda suggests a number of herbs for the treatment of such disorders, it recommends more rest and a lighter diet to reduce physical and emotional discomfort.

Ashoka

Ashoka is a premium ayurvedic herb for treating almost any kind of gynecological problem known to womankind. A sacred tree of immense literary significance, ashoka literally translates as "without sorrow." The ashoka tree appears in many ancient texts as the reliever of women's pain and a friend of women. The powder extracted from the tree bark is extensively used in ayurvedic medicines for helping with many genito-urinary conditions.

Ashoka has been traditionally used in irregular periods, missing periods, excessive bleeding, painful periods, prolonged periods, and hormonal imbalances, as well as in PMS symptoms like irritability, mood swings, fever, nausea, bloating, or indigestion. The high iron and calcium content of ashoka prevents anemia due to heavy blood loss and helps with fatigue, weakness, dizziness, and headaches. According to a 2014 study, ashoka is rich in saponins, flavonoids, glycosides, tannins, essential oils, iron, and calcium that altogether act as a tonic for the uterine muscles. However, strictly avoid taking ashoka during pregnancy, as it is also used to induce labor pain.

Shatavari

Shatavari is a versatile female tonic used to enhance beauty and wellness. Shatavari literally translates as "the one with a thousand husbands," signifying its ability to strengthen female reproductive organs. Its powerful antispasmodic property prevents contractions of uterine muscles and reduces the risk of abdominal cramps. Regular use can calm hormonal imbalances and help with irregular periods, heavy bleeding, irritability, and mood swings. Shatavari is also an excellent uterine tonic and a powerful internal moisturizer that protects vaginal tissues against infections, dryness, and pathogens.

Shatavari is also known for its immense mental health benefits. Classified as a rasayana (rejuvenating) herb in ayurveda, shatavari is traditionally used to reduce stress, enhance immunity, improve sleep quality, and help with mental disorders. It is also completely safe during pregnancy, and, in fact, protects the fetus from miscarriage risks.

Ajwain (carom seeds) + methi seeds (fenugreek) + gud (jaggery)

A mix of jaggery, methi, and ajwain is very effective in dealing with a range of muscular tension and abdominal cramps. Prepare small-size balls with these three ingredients and take two to three of these on an empty stomach with lukewarm water.

Unripe Papaya

Green, unripe papaya is considered useful in strengthening muscle fibers in the uterus and regulating menstrual flow. Drink the juice of unripe papaya regularly for a few weeks for a healthy uterus.

Aloe Vera

Aloe vera helps to manage menstrual irregularities naturally by regulating the hormonal disorder, both in the case of dysmenorrhea and amenorrhea (avoid this remedy during periods). Aloe vera is rich because it gives B complex vitamin to the body, which regulates the pH of the stomach and reduces fat. Consume aloe vera juice mixed with one teaspoon of honey before having breakfast.

Ginger and Turmeric

Ginger and turmeric are the most commonly prescribed herbs for pain associated with menstrual cycles and are quite warming as well. Turmeric and ginger are considered to be the best-medicated herbs and helpful in regulating menstruation and balancing hormones. The antispasmodic and anti-inflammatory properties support in balancing hormones and relieving menstrual pain. The patient may consume two teaspoons of ginger juice or one-quarter teaspoon of turmeric with lukewarm water.

Yoga Therapy for Menstrual Disorders

Menstrual disorders are very common for most women which arise due to a physical or emotional problem that interferes with a normal menstrual cycle. It brings a lot of stress to both the patients and their parents. Here yoga plays an important role by improving the functioning of the endocrine glands, which regulates the menstruation. Yoga not only promotes flexibility, the muscles become supple and do not cramp, but also the stress level which is a major cause of these disorders decreases. Regular practice of yoga and living a natural life is essential for every patient to control and cure menstrual disorders.

Yoga therapy techniques like dhauti and basti can detoxify the body and remove all ama (toxins) from the body and rejuvenate the system. Kapalabhati kriya should be avoided during the menstruation time.

The main yoga practices for treating the menstruation disorders are yoga breathing exercises, warm-up exercises, surya namaskar followed by savasana, at least five sittings, prone and supine yoga asanas daily, pranayama, and meditation.

Breathing and warm-up exercises, surya namaskar and yoga asanas should be done very slowly and carefully during the menstruation times and normal speed before and after the periods. Nadi shuddhi pranayama two times daily , morning and evening, on an empty stomach, about nine rounds in each session, followed by fifteen to thirty minutes of meditation can bring complete recovery of the menstruation problems over two to three months. Yoga nidra for thirty minutes or more can be practiced at the end of daily yoga sessions to reverse menstruation complications and painful menstruation. Practice yoni mudra (yoni means 'womb', and mudra refers to hand posture), a type of mudra yoga, one hour daily during the menstruation times, which can reduce the pain and complications of menstruation.

The following processes are very useful for the control and cure of the troubles discussed above. However, it is good to practice pranayama, yoga nidra, and savasana while bleeding is going on, and also to avoid practicing many other asanas.

Yoga Nidra

It is an excellent practice as useful in all diseases. The regular practice of yoga nidra is helpful to overcome the psychiatric morbidity associated with menstrual irregularities. Therefore, yogic relaxation training like yoga nidra is highly effective to control stress and pain related to menstrual dysfunction.

Surya Namaskar (Sun Salutation)

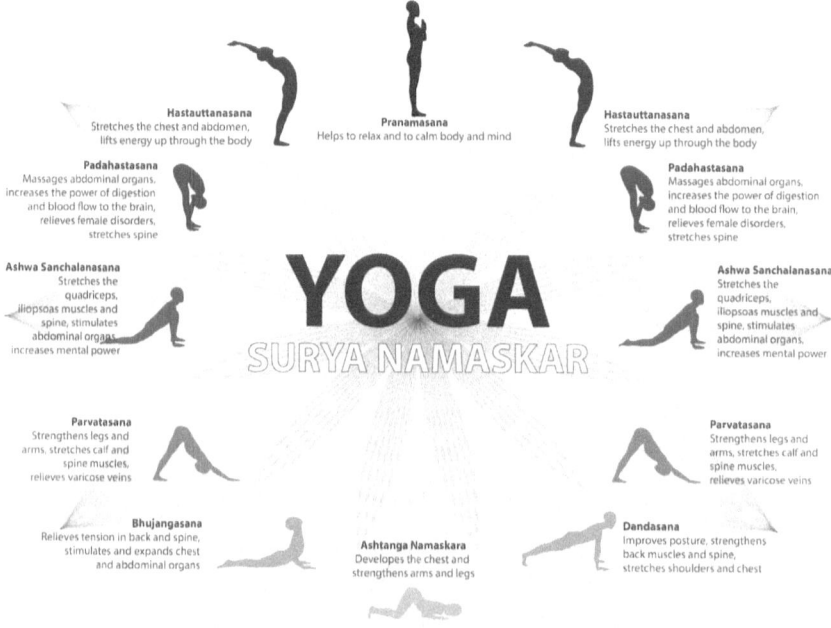

Sun Salutation is a comprehensive exercise, a series of asanas helpful for strengthening overall body function and to treat this problem. Just like asanas, the patient needs to perform sun salutation slowly and with supportive breathing techniques.

Asanas (Yoga Poses)

- **Bhujangasana (cobra pose)**

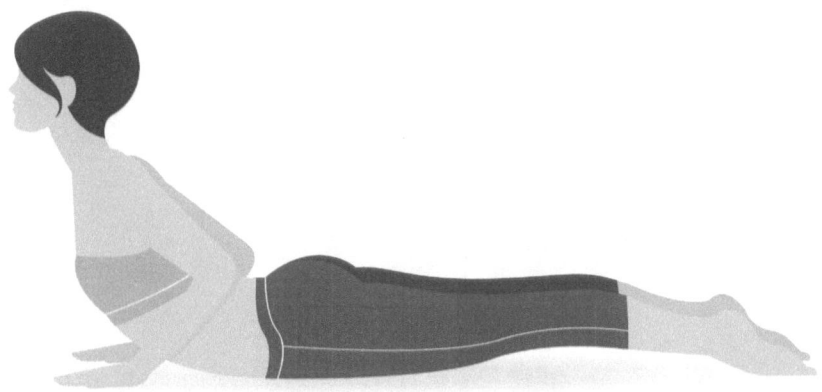

It is an excellent yoga asana for stimulating reproductive organs. It improves blood circulation in the body by activating core muscles. The cobra pose is a great help for relieving menstrual pain as it reduces fatigue and stress.

- Lie down on your chest (in prone position), face down.
- Feet hip-width apart and the top of your feet flat on the floor with your toes spread.
- Place your palms slightly lower than your shoulder, with the tips of your fingers right below your shoulder muscles and elbows close to your body pointing behind you and not outward.
- Inhale as you slowly lift your head and chest off the ground. Pull your shoulders back and your chest forward, but do not crunch your neck. Keep your shoulders away from your ears and bring their gaze up to the ceiling, your arms bent at your elbows.
- Feel your stomach pressed on the ground and stay in this position with normal breathing for one minute.
- To release the pose, slowly bring your body down part by part until your forehead touches the ground. Then, place your hands

under your head and rest your head on one side and breathe normally.

- **Dhanurasana (bow pose)**

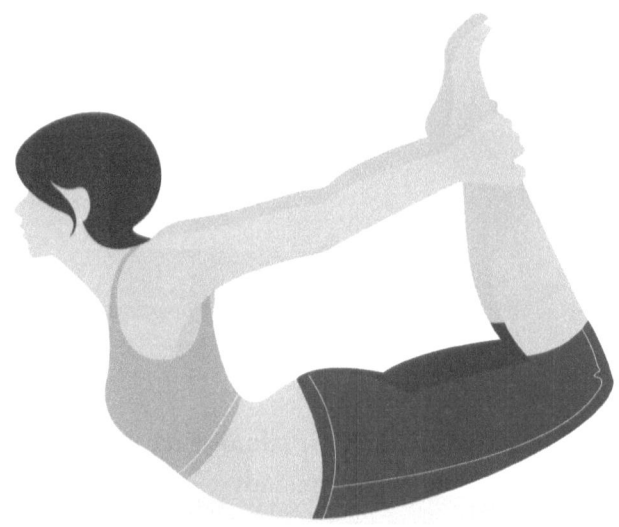

The bow pose strengthens the abdominal muscles and stimulates the groin region. Improves digestion and appetite, cures dyspepsia (obesity), and gastrointestinal problems. It is helpful to alleviate menstrual discomfort and constipation.

- Lie down on your chest (in prone position), face down.
- Bend your knees and use your hands to grab your ankles.
- As you inhale, lift your shoulders, chest, and thighs off the ground. Slowly pull your legs outward and backward so that your spine is arched like a bow.
- Rest on your abdomen and do not bend your elbows.
- Gaze forward and hold the pose for about thirty seconds while focusing on stretching, balancing and breathing. Do not hold your breath.

- To release the pose, exhale and slowly lower down your thighs, chest, and shoulders on the ground. Let go of your ankles and place your hands by the side of your body.
- Rest with either side of your ear on the mat. Relax for a few seconds and repeat the pose as needed.

- **Baddha konasana (cobbler's pose)**

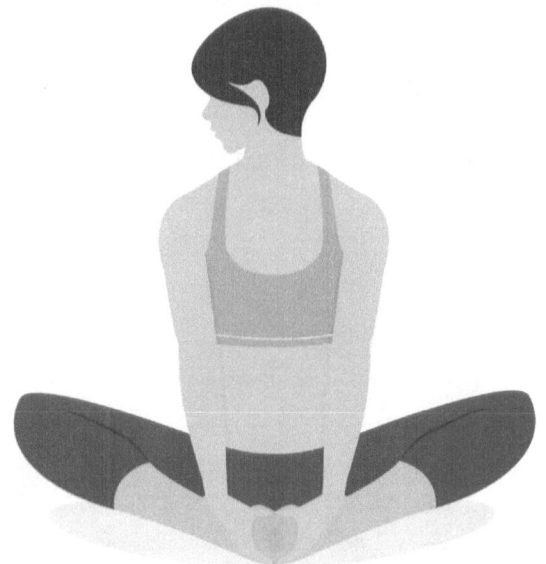

It opens the pelvic region, groin area, and hip joint. This asana helps to relieve urinary disorders, regulates the menstrual flow, and rejuvenates the kidneys, bladder, and prostate gland. It is one of the best poses for pregnant women in preparation for childbirth. The patient may feel more relaxed by bending forward using a bolster or a folded blanket to support the torso.

- Sit in dandasana (staff pose) with your legs stretched out straight in front of you.
- Now bend your knees and bring the soles of your feet together.

- Hold your feet and ankles as you let your knees fall out to both sides.
- Draw your heels in as close to your groin. Back off if you feel any pain or discomfort.
- Sit up tall with a long spine. Your arms and shoulders should be relaxed.
- Press the sitting bones on the floor and let the crown of the head point toward the ceiling to elongate the spine.
- Hold this pose for up to two minutes or so.
- To release from the pose, return to dandasana (staff pose).

- **Paschimottanasana (seated forward bend)**

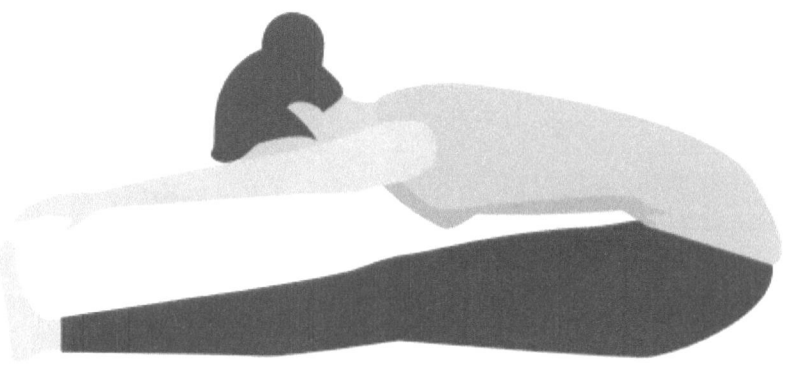

This advanced forward bend asana is yet another yoga pose that massages the abdominal organs, back muscles, groin area, and the whole body, thus alleviating pain caused by menstrual cramps.

- Sit in dandasana (staff pose) with your legs stretched out straight in front of you.
- Keep your spine erect and toes pointing toward you.
- Inhale and gently raise both arms straight above your head and stretch up.

- As you exhale, slowly bend your trunk forward from the hip joint, chin moving toward the toes, keeping the spine erect. Arm stretched and hands parallel to the ground.
- If possible, catch hold of your toes and pull them to help you bend forward farther until your trunk and face rest on your knees. Do not bend your knees.
- Bend your hands at the elbow and relax your abdominal muscles.
- Stay in this position for about a minute with normal breathing.
- After one minute, inhale and slowly raise up your arms straight above your head.
- Then at exhalation, bring your arms down, placing the palms on the ground.
- Relax for a while in dandasana and observe the changes that occurred in the body.

- **Ushtrasana (camel pose)**

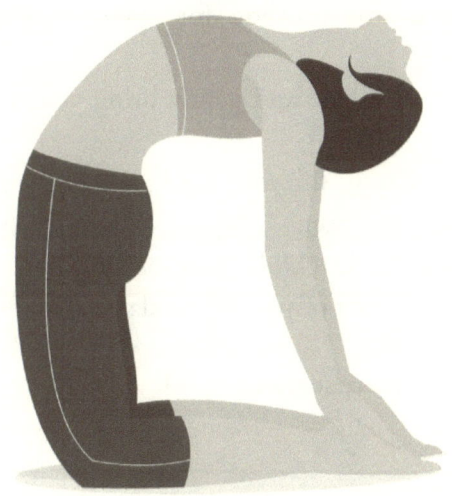

This camel pose is another excellent pose that provides complete stretch and stimulates reproductive organs and brings great relief to menstrual pain/discomfort.

- Sit on your heels, stretching your lower legs backward and keeping them together.
- Now, stand on your knees with your legs hip-width apart.
- Place your hands on your hips to support your back, fingers pointing forward, and your thumbs resting on your lower back facing toward each other. The elbows should be pointing behind.
- Keep your hips over your knees in one line.
- Now, as you inhale, round your shoulders back and open your chest. Then with an exhalation, push your hips forward and slowly bend your spine backward from the waist.
- Once you feel stable, bring your palms down to your ankles of your feet, one by one.
- Maintain this position for about a minute with normal breathing.
- To release, inhale and gently bring your hands on the lower back one by one.
- Simultaneously, lift your head and chest up and come back to the initial position.
- You can rest in child's pose or simply stretch your legs out straight in front of you (in dandasana) and relax.

- **Savasana (corpse pose)**

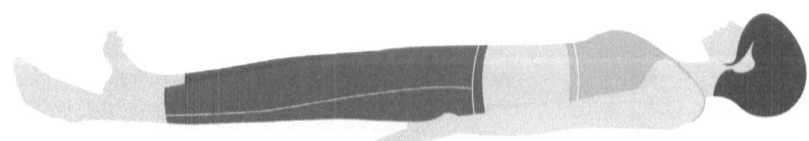

Savasana is an important pose for every woman suffering from menstrual disorders, as it helps to release stress, tension, fatigue, anxiety, and depression.

— Lie down on your back. Feet apart, arms alongside your body, turn your palms upward facing toward the ceiling. Collapse your whole body, soften your facial muscles, and make a beautiful smile.
— Close your eyes and observe your whole body from your toes all the way up to the head.
— Now, at each inhalation and exhalation, relax your body part by part, starting from your lower part (toes to hips), then shift your awareness to the upper part (from your abdomen to your neck), and finally your head region.
— Stay in this position for about ten minutes while observing the changes throughout your body.

Pranayama

Pranayama are more useful techniques than asanas to get rid of menstrual disorders. A patient of the menstrual disorder can reduce the stress, balance the emotions, and calm the mind with the regular practice of pranayama. Anuloma-viloma, ujjayi, and bhramari pranayama are most beneficial for these disorders.

Tips to practice pranayama

• Pranayama should be practiced peacefully and without any jerk.
• Slow and deep breathing is very much beneficial.
• The patient should practice without breath holding (kumbhak) and bandhas (breathe locking) techniques.
• Avoid pranayama, which will generate excess heat in the body like fast breathing, bhastrika (bellows breath), surya bhedan (right nostril breathing), and kapalbhati (frontal brain cleansing).

Naturopathic therapy

From age to age and from region to region, it's rare to find a woman with a symptom-free menstrual cycle. Naturopathy plays an important role to control and manage the menstrual disorders such as cramping, pain, excessive bleeding, irregular bleeding, and uncontrollable moods and helps to live a happy life.

Naturopathy recommends:

- Include milk and plenty of fruit to your breakfast (sprouted beans, milk, buttermilk, tomato, carrot, orange, sweet lime, banana, pineapple, apple, figs, almonds, coconut water).
- Lunch and dinner should consist of wholemeal bread and boiled vegetables.
- Increase intake of water, drink at least two to three liters of water in the day.
- Fasting once in a week (with only lemon juice and water).
- Yoga, meditation, walking, and light exercises should be done/ practiced regularly.
- Avoid all kinds of fried, spicy, and sour food.

Conclusions

Painful menstruation, absence of menstruation, and excessive bleeding during menses is an abnormal state that arises due to stress, anxiety, the wrong type of diet, and an unnatural way of living. Problems like constipation and, in some cases, dysmenorrhoea develop because of too much addiction to tea and painkiller to relieve the headache, addiction to refined and fried foods, and lack of exercise.

Every patient needs to take an adequate amount of water throughout the day. The patient should give up processed foods, polished rice, a high amount of sugar, and tea. Other than the above-mentioned techniques, regular practice of yoga and living a natural life is essential for every patient to control and cure menstrual disorders.

Chapter 5

Healing Digestive Disorders

Foods that we ingest are the chief source of fulfilling the required energy for our body to sustain and grow. So a clear understanding of the digestive processes that go on in the human body is vital to understand the disorders from which digestion suffers. The incorporation of food in the human body is accomplished by a threefold process of digestion, absorption, and assimilation. Digestion begins the moment food enters the mouth. It mixes with the saliva and is made more permeable for the gastric juice, which exudes from the openings of the tiny glands of the stomach. The churning of the stomach mixes the food with the gastric juices and hydrochloric acid and when it becomes soluble, it passes to the intestines and at last into the bowel. The more light the food, the easier it is digested.

When the food passes into the intestine, it is exposed to the action of bile, pancreatic juices, intestinal juice, and the bacteria. These juices contain elements that break down the food into products like glycerine, which sustains the system. Food materials are absorbed almost exclusively by the small intestine, water, and salt through the large intestine. The indigestible residue, alongside various substances which are waste, excreted from the liver and therefore the intestinal walls, is thrown out of the body within the stools.

Assimilation is a much slower process. The blood circulates through every organ and takes from it what's necessary for its own growth and repair. The cells within the bones extract lime salts, muscles sugar, and protein. The greater bulk is assimilated by the muscles.

Causes of Digestive Disorders

Indigestion or dyspepsia is the elemental digestive disorder that can produce more acute or serious diseases in the later stage. The basic reason for indigestion, besides weak digestive powers, is overeating or eating wrong foods that are not suitable for our body. Feces of such persons contain large amounts of undigested matter, and they suffer from flatulence arising from the putrefying matter in the stomach or the intestines. Such a situation develops functional digestive disorders like a feeling of fullness amounting to heaviness, loss of appetite, and general discomfort.

Common Digestive Disorders

Acidity, also called acid reflux, is a result of an increase in the quantity of acid released into the stomach. Mental stress, rich diet, today's lifestyle, and bad habits are the major causes of this acidity production. A person of such conditions can suffer from burning sensation in the chest, and pain.

Chronic Diarrhea

Diarrhea is a common condition and a key symptom in many disorders like irritable bowel syndrome. It happens mainly due to virus or sometimes contaminated food.

Constipation

Constipation is a trouble experienced by people of all age groups. However, not many are aware that it is an intimation of an impaired body system, inflammatory bowel disease (IBD), or colon cancer.

Colitis

It is a serious disease of the colon. The disease occurs due to a specific virus that swells the large intestine, impairing its function and causing frequent diarrhea.

Peptic Ulcer

Prolonged trouble of acidity damages the lining of the intestine and eventually causes injury to the digestive tract. As the sore goes deeper and deeper, it produces a hole into the intestine, which, if left untreated, could be fatal. This is known as a stomach ulcer.

Haemorrhoids

Also called piles, these are swollen veins inside the anus and lower rectum. Regular eating of oily and rich food, obesity, and constipation are the major cause of developing haemorrhoids.

Ayurvedic Therapy

The importance of digestion for overall wellness cannot be overemphasized. Poor digestion can not only lower the quality of life on a day-to-day basis but affects immunity, sleep, and almost every aspect of physical and emotional health. Ayurveda recognizes healthy digestion as one of the most fundamental aspects of wellness.

Digestion is recognized as the key to perfect health and the root cause of all diseases.

There are three pillars of health in ayurveda: proper digestion, healthful sleep, and right management of sexuality—with digestion being the foremost for the proper working of immune function. Good digestion is not only desirable; it's a precondition for leading a healthy and productive life.

You are not only what you eat, but when you eat, how you eat, and—the most important of all—how you digest it.

The food we eat gets mixed with enzymes and acids, and the end product is called the ahara ras (the essence of food), which is used to make tissues. Complete digestion takes into account the breaking down of food matter, conversion to ahara ras, absorption, as well as assimilation of nutrients in the body.

Digestion is important because this essence of food is what provides the body its physical form. In fact, diet is a profound aspect of ayurvedic healing. Ayurvedic therapies rely so much on dietary interventions that digestion in itself becomes a prerequisite for enabling the innate healing potential of the human body.

Digestion is a holistic concept in the ayurvedic philosophy. Mental digestion of newly acquired information, ideas, emotions, experiences, and interactions with other people is as important as the physical digestion of food. Nonetheless, we will limit our discussion to the physical aspect of digestion.

Just as the healthy digestion of food is essential for a healthy body, digestion of experiences is crucial for a healthy mind.

Agni – the Flame of Digestion

The fire energy, also known as the digestive flame (agni), is responsible for governing all the metabolic processes in the body. The quality of digestion depends on the quality of this digestive flame. Agni can be understood as the strength of digestive juices. An overactive flame may burn everything and result in wastage of nutrients, whereas a low flame will result in incomplete digestion of food and accumulation of toxins over time.

Constipation, bloating, gas, and headaches are manifestations of a weak flame, a condition where the process is too slow because of inadequate action of enzymes. On the other hand, diarrhea, acid reflux, hyperacidity, heartburn, and dyspepsia are a result of too quick digestion—a manifestation of overactive flame. Ayurvedic way of life strives to maintain an optimal digestive flame through conscious eating, regular eating habits, meditation, yoga, and various other lifestyle adaptations.

1. Get the right spices

To enhance the digestive flame, adding some spices to the diet is recommended. Pungent spices like ginger, black pepper, cumin seeds, garlic, or cayenne are great for increasing the flame. Spices stimulate the secretion of digestive juices that help in the breakdown of food matter. However, spices should always be used in moderation as too much of spices can give you acid reflux. Also, some people are already blessed with a good digestive flame and do not require additional support.

For people who experience frequent heartburn symptoms after eating, consider reducing pungent foods and replace them with astringent spices, such as saffron, turmeric, basil, oregano, or coriander. Astringent, bitter, and sweet tastes help in calming an overactive flame, therefore helping with hyperacidity and indigestion. Salty, sour, and pungent tastes can help with low flame conditions like chronic constipation or gas.

2. Kindle the fire energy

Adding some sour foods like yogurt or buttermilk can help increase the flame, therefore stimulating the organs and helping in easy digestion. However, avoid sour foods during the summer season. Protecting the flame is another aspect of aiding the natural digestion process. Drinking cold water with meals or just before meals can harm the fire energy and dilute the strength of digestive juices.

This is why ayurveda advises against drinking too much water while eating. Alcohol and caffeinated beverages are also considered harmful for the digestive fire. Instead, sip warm water or water at room temperature. Also, try to drink plenty of water throughout the day to help absorption and assimilation of nutrients. Water helps in the natural detoxification process, therefore reducing the risk of waste accumulation.

3. Consistent meals

Irregular or skipped meals can harm the rhythmic working of the fire energy. While ayurveda recommends fasting between seasons to cleanse the digestive organs, it advises against unplanned fasting. Eat regular meals at fixed intervals and try to eat at the same time every day to establish a routine. Irregularity and indiscipline in any sphere of life can imbalance the vata dosha, aggravation of which is responsible for constipation, poor transfer of nutrients, and brain fog.

4. Eat six tastes at every meal

Ayurveda recognizes six kinds of tastes: sweet, sour, salty, astringent, bitter, and pungent. Each taste stimulates a particular organ and has some positive and negative effects on all the three doshas. For example, the sweet taste is favorable for vata and pitta but is harmful to kapha. Pungent taste pacifies kapha but aggravates both vata and pitta. Eating all the six tastes at every meal is important because taken together, their effects cancel out each other and the balance is maintained. Also, consuming all the six tastes can help in satisfying the taste buds, enabling the mind to derive maximum gratification from the food.

Ayurvedic Remedies for Digestive Disorders

As per medical studies, more or less five out of ten people suffer from digestion problems like gas, bloating, stomach pain, constipation, heartburn, and fatigue after eating. Ayurveda provides simple, easy-to-practice and straightforward solutions to those common problems.

Cleansing the complete digestive system includes virechana, using some purgative herbs or oils, and cleaning the entire system from mouth to the rectum. Hot water mixed with lemon juice can also clean the system.

Like yoga therapy, ayurveda also uses dhauti and basti (Vasti) for the removal of ama from the digestive tract through the stomach and small and large intestines and expelled through the anus. Massage techniques like panchakarma and abhyanga , and rejuvenating techniques of shirodhara like thakra dhara are also adopted for removing ama from the system to rejuvenate the brain and nervous system.

These treatments will eliminate the emotional, mental, and physical ama (toxins) from the system and create digestive enzymes with the introduction of naturally soft and smooth liquid foods.

Constipation is caused by a vata imbalance. Therefore, consuming a vata-balancing diet is the best way to treat constipation. Ayurveda recommends a mixture of hot water, ghee, and salt for a quick fix for constipation.

Ripened papaya is the ultimate solution for all digestive disorders! Eat papaya daily thirty minutes before or one hour after lunch, which can cure all digestive disorders, including stomach cancer. The enzyme papain in papaya has the power to cure even cancer!

Another important remedy for digestive problems like peptic ulcer, mouth ulcer, stomach ulcer is to drink ash gourd juice or eat fresh pieces daily every morning on an empty stomach or one hour after breakfast and lunch. This will balance all pitta imbalance and make the body and mind calm and healthy.

Drinks that can help to cleanse the complete digestive system includes:

- **Triphala powder (hirda, behda, and amla)**

Drink one teaspoon + one glass of lukewarm water nightly before getting to bed.

- **Dried black grapes**

Soak 40-50 gm of dried black grapes in one glass of cold water at night. Eat them in the morning, and drink the water in which they were soaked.

- **Amla + Ginger**

Mix amla powder (25 gm) + two teaspoons of ginger juice + two teaspoons of honey and take the combination early in the morning with an empty stomach.

- **Nisoth**

Also referred to as turpeth root, it is a useful herb for conditions like indigestion or constipation. Drink nisoth juice with a glass of water every morning on an empty stomach. It will help to manage and to scale back the danger of gastric ulcers, hyperacidity, and indigestion.

Yoga Therapy for Digestive Disorders

Shat kriya techniques are the first way to heal digestive disorders. Mainly jala neti and trataka cleanse the nasal and ocular ama and balance the ajna chakra by eliminating the mental and emotional ama from the system. Vastra dhauti , vamana dhauti , and shanka prakshalana cleanse the digestive system for the restoration of the digestive processes and rejuvenation of jatharagni (digestive fire). The practice of agnisara followed by nauli weekly can improve the quality of jatharagni in the belly. One who practices agnisara and nauli once in a week will have pure and high jatharagni and good digestive power. Kapalabhati kriya also increases jatharagni.

The practice of nadi shuddhi pranayama three times a day with nine rounds in every session, followed by fifteen or thirty minutes of meditation for a period of one or two months can heal any type of digestive disorder. Along with this, bhramari and ujjayi pranayama can improve the quality of sleep, which induces high jatharagni , and proper digestive functions.

Yogic Kriyas

Agnisar

It is one of the best and easy techniques to burn toxins and to strengthen the digestive organs for better digestion. Other than the digestive system, this yogic exercise also stimulates the immune system, circulatory system, and increases the heat in the body.

- Stand with your feet about six inches apart. Lean your upper body forward from the waist, rest your palms on your thighs with your arms straight and keep your back relaxed.
- As you exhale through your mouth, vigorously contract the muscles in the lower abdomen and the area above the pelvis and suck them inward and upward toward the spine.
- Then inhale, and gently release the muscles, allowing the lower abdomen to relax and return to its natural position.
- Repeat with this pumping in and out movement for as many times as you can.
- Once finished, come up to tadasana (standing position) and relax with normal breathing.

It is best practiced when the stomach and bowels are empty, typically early in the morning.

Vaman Dhauti

Vaman dhauti is meant for purification of the upper digestive tract, i.e., the mouth, teeth, stomach, and intestines. It helps to remove gas, acidity, and extra mucus from the food pipe.

- Prepare about one and a half liter of warm water and add in two tablespoons of salt. Stir well until salt dissolves.
- Drink the saline water as quickly as you can until your stomach can't contain it anymore and you feel the urge to vomit.

- Now slowly churn your stomach by doing twisting movements until you are able to vomit out all the water.
- If you are unable to vomit, insert the middle three fingers of your right hand and tickle the back of your throat until you vomit out all the water. Repeat tickling the throat until no more water comes out.
- Once completed, relax completely in savasana for about fifteen minutes.
- After half an hour, have a bland and light breakfast. Try to avoid spicy food, coffee, and tea during the first three hours after vaman dhauti.

This is to be done early in the morning on empty stomach and bowels are empty.

Asanas (Yoga Poses)

- **Vajrasana (thunderbolt pose)**

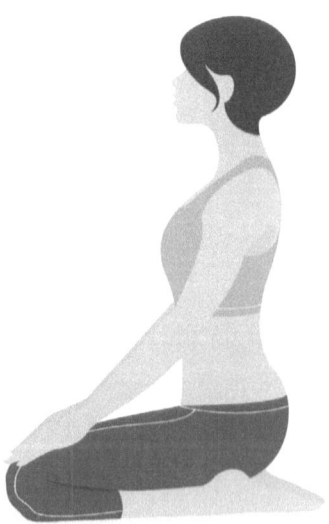

Vajrasana, also known as thunderbolt pose, is one of the easiest yoga asanas to perform. It can be performed at any point in time even after the meal. This position improves blood circulation in the abdominal region, which is essential for digestion.

- Kneel down and keep your lower legs together. Try to bring your big toes and heels as close as possible. If you have stiff ankles, roll a towel underneath to support the joint and arch of ankles.
- Gently rest your buttocks your heels and your thighs on your calf muscles.
- Then place your hands on your knees and set your gaze forward, keeping your head straight.
- Now focus on your breath and observe your breathing pattern, how you inhale and exhale.
- You may close your eyes for good concentration of your breathing and to calm your mind.
- Stay in this position for at least five to ten minutes.

- **Pawanmuktasana (wind-relieving pose)**

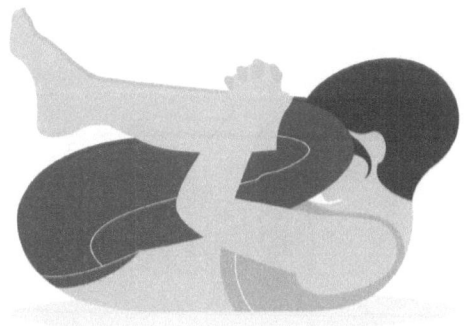

This asana is specifically designed in easing bloating and gastric troubles. It strengthens the intestines and internal organs by giving a good massage to the abdominal area, therefore, helping to release trapped gases and improves digestion. Those who are suffering from piles should avoid this asana.

- Lie down on your back with your feet together and arms by the side of your body.
- Inhale and as you exhale, draw both knee toward your chest and press your thigh against your abdomen with clasped hands.
- Inhale again and as you exhale, lift your head and chest off the ground and bring your chin on your knees.
- Stay in this position as long as possible with deep, long breaths in and out.
- Inhale and as you exhale, bring both hands down by the side of your body and slowly lower down your legs one by one on the ground and rest in the supine position.
- Repeat for another three to five times.

- **Uttanpadasana (leg raised)**

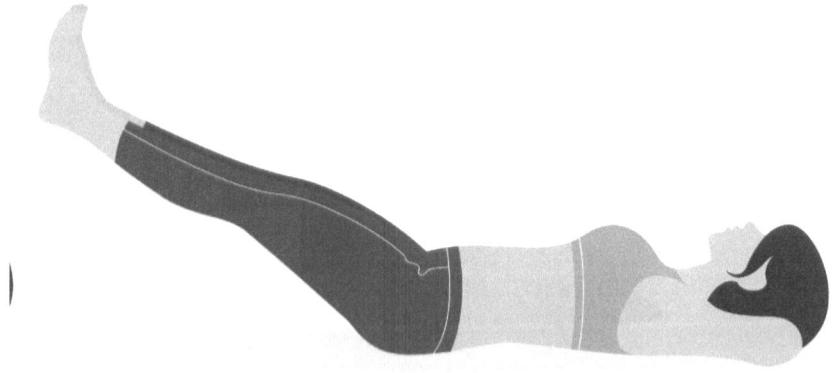

It generates acute pressure and improves the tone and strength of the abdominal muscles. Regular practice of this asana can cure stomach disorders like acidity, indigestion, and constipation.

- Lie down comfortably on your back in supine position, feet together and arms by the side of your body with your palms facing downward. Relax your whole body and breathe normally.
- Inhale and slowly raise both legs up to an angle of about 45 degrees from the ground without bending the knees while raising your legs.
- Stay in this position for as long as you can, and while maintaining, inhale and exhale slowly.
- To release from the pose, exhale and bring down your legs slowly.
- Repeat for another three to five rounds.

A lot of pressure can be felt at the abdominal muscles, and if you feel strain at the abdomen, lower the legs and relax for a few seconds

- **Paschimottanasana (seated forward bend)**

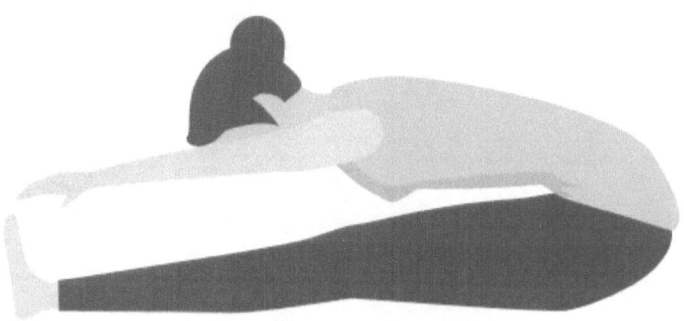

This advanced asana is helpful to control and cure many digestive disorders. It improves the flexibility and strength of all major organs of the body such as spinal cord, liver, kidneys, stomach, pancreas, and intestines, which are helpful for proper digestion.

- Sit in dandasana (staff pose) with your legs stretched out straight in front of you.

- Keep your spine erect and toes pointing toward you.
- Inhale and gently raise both arms straight above your head and stretch up.
- As you exhale, slowly bend your trunk forward from the hip joint, chin moving toward the toes, keeping the spine erect. Arm stretched and hands parallel to the ground.
- If possible, catch hold of your toes and pull them to help you bend forward farther until your trunk and face rest on your knees. Do not bend your knees.
- Bend your hands at the elbow and relax your abdominal muscles.
- Stay in this position for about a minute with normal breathing.
- After one minute, inhale and slowly raise up your arms straight above your head.
- Then at exhalation, bring your arms down, placing the palms on the ground.
- Relax for a while in dandasana and observe the changes that occurred in the body.

- **Ardha naukasana (half-boat pose)**

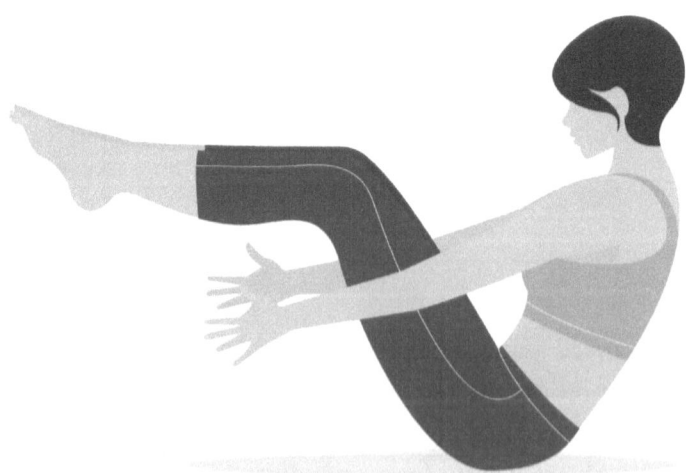

One of the most well-known and interesting yoga poses deeply challenges the abdominal region. It improves the strength of the core muscles, kidneys, prostate glands, and intestines and thus helpful for the smooth digestion process.

— Sit on the floor with your legs stretched out in front of you, hands by the sides with your palms on the ground.
— Bend your knees and keep your feet firmly on the ground.
— Lift your chest up and lean back, and try to keep your spine erect.
— Inhale and lift your feet up to the knee height. Ensure that the calf muscles are parallel to the ground and thighs remain perpendicular.
— Then slowly, lift your arms parallel to the floor close to your body and your palms facing each other.
— Feel the tension at your navel area as the abdominal muscles contract.
— Continue breathing deeply while maintaining this position steadily for as long as you can.
— To release, exhale slowly as you bring your hands and legs down to the starting position and relax.
— Repeat for three to five times but do not overdo it.

Pranayama

- **Kapalabhati (skull-shining breathing)**

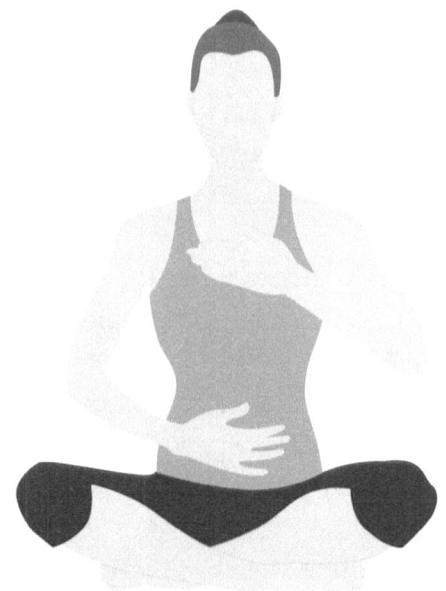

It improves the function of the pancreas, liver, kidney, and intestine, and helps to supply insulin and other digestive hormones naturally. Calms the mind and removes toxins from the interior system. A patient with digestive disorders must practice kapalabhati pranayama at low or moderate speed. The regular practice of kapalabhati and a balanced diet brings excellent results for problems associated with the gastrointestinal system. People who suffer from cardiac problems, hypertension, and hernia and spinal disorders are to avoid this practice.

- Sit comfortably in any meditative position with your spine and neck erect.
- Place your hands on your knees with palms facing downward.
- Inhale passively through your nostrils, and as you exhale forcefully and quickly, pull your belly in all the way back toward the spine.

– Repeat the forceful exhalation as quickly as you can at the rate of 60 contractions per minute.

– You may place one hand on the stomach to feel the contraction of your abdominal muscles and one on your chest.

– After completion of the first round, inhale deeply through your nostrils, and exhale slowly through your mouth.

– Relax with your eyes closed and observe your breath and the sensations throughout your body.

– When your breathing is back to normal, slowly open your eyes.

– You may repeat another one or two rounds.

Meditation for Digestion

Digestion may be a natural action, but stress and anxiety create a negative impact on biological processes, especially digestion. Guided meditation programs, while focusing the mind to the navel center, will yield many great benefits to enhance digestive disorders. Deep meditation helps to scale back stress and anxiety, improves blood circulation within the body, and relieves many disorders connected to the stomach and intestines.

Naturopathic Therapy

Naturopathy strongly advocates that gut health is often restored with healthy eating and right living habits. It's possible that a perfect diet, regular exercise, and stress-free life will control and cure many health disorders, especially digestion problems.

Naturopathy recommends:

- The cardinal remedy for the digestive disorder is light food, which is definitely digestible.
- Masticate your food properly so that it mixes well with the saliva.
- Bland food, mostly vegetables cooked in water, juicy fruits, and buttermilk (churned curd with water added), should be taken.
- Sleep on the left side for ten to fifteen minutes after meals.
- Do not drink water during meals. Instead, drink water one hour after meals.
- Have a mix of one glass lukewarm water and half lemon juice on an empty stomach in the morning.
- Eat ripe papaya (little in quantity) with black pepper and halite to enhance digestion.
- Drink a minimum of three liters of water throughout the day.

Conclusions

All disease begins within the gut. Patients can get permanent relief if they increase their body heat through regular exercise. Indigestion may be a sedentary disease; active and brisk people generally don't suffer from this malady.

Alcohol, tobacco, and rich and spicy food should be avoided or should be taken within the minimum possible quantity. Strengthen the system—eat many plants (fruits and vegetables; the more polyphenol-rich, the better), drink enough water, do yoga each day, get daily distressing time and restful sleep because our digestive health is tied to immune function.

Chapter 6

Healing Respiratory Disorders

Respiratory diseases are a variety of pathogenic conditions that affect the airways and other structures of the lung. Respiration is the process of exchanging gas and involves taking oxygen into the body and expelling carbon dioxide from the body. Respiratory disease is known as pulmonology and occurs in the respiratory tract, including the alveoli, bronchi, bronchioles, pleura, pleural cavity, trachea, and the nerves and muscles of respiration.

As per medical science, respiratory diseases can be classified in many different ways, but there are three main types of respiratory diseases: airway diseases, lung tissue diseases, and lung circulation diseases. Airway diseases limit the amount of air that is able to enter alveoli because of blockage in the passageways. Asthma, COPD, and bronchiectasis are coming under airway diseases. Lung tissue diseases affect the structure of lung tissue and make the lungs unable to expand fully.

A patient of such condition feels difficult to take in oxygen and release carbon dioxide due to inflammation of the lung tissue. Pulmonary fibrosis and sarcoidosis are few examples of restrictive lung disease or lung tissue disease. Lung circulation diseases are the condition where the blood vessels in the lungs affect due to clotting, scarring, or inflammation. These diseases seriously affect the functioning of the heart and the ability of the lungs to receive oxygen and produce carbon dioxide.

The most common lung diseases are:

Asthma

Asthma is a chronic noncommunicable disease of the lungs. This condition arises when the airways are constantly inflamed, causing wheezing and recurrent attacks of breathlessness. Depending on the person, asthma symptoms may become worse at night and may occur a few times a day or a few times per week. Allergies, sinus infections, pollution, tobacco smoking, breathing in some chemicals, physical exercise, and bad weather can trigger asthma symptoms. According to a WHO report, more than 250 million people currently suffer from asthma and it is a common disease among children.

COPD

Chronic obstructive pulmonary disease (COPD), which includes emphysema and chronic bronchitis, makes the bronchial tubes (the air passages between the mouth nose, and lungs) hard to breathe. COPD can limit the ability to perform simple daily tasks for the patient. The symptoms and treatment are different from person to person and there is no "best" medicine for all people to cure COPD.

Nasal allergy (allergic rhinitis)

Nasal allergy, also called allergic rhinitis, is a harmless health problem that causes an allergic reaction in the respiratory system. This problem may be seasonal or perennial. Mostly, an allergen-like pollen causes an allergic reaction in our body, which is what we call allergic rhinitis or hay fever. Cigarette smoke, chemicals, cold temperatures, humidity, and air pollution can trigger nasal allergies. Unfortunately, in the long run, allergic rhinitis may develop certain complications such as sleeping disorder, development of asthma symptoms, frequent ear infections, and frequent sinus infections.

Ayurvedic Therapy for Respiratory Disorders

In ayurveda, respiratory disorders are primarily a result of kapha and vata aggravation. Excess vata can increase the dryness in the lungs and cause infections, shortness of breath, chest pain, asthma, or allergies. Kapha aggravation causes excess mucus production in the body, which moves to the lungs, thickens, and blocks respiratory pathways. Excess kapha can cause sinusitis, bronchitis, asthma, pneumonia, and worsen allergies and cough problems.

Kapha-vata aggravation, coupled with excess pitta, can also cause inflammation of respiratory pathways and worsen these symptoms. Low digestive fire is another reason for respiratory disorders, as incomplete digestion can cause accumulation of mucus, which then moves to the lungs and causes congestions. Improper breathing, extremely dry and rough weather (like winter or autumn), environmental pollutants, unplanned fasting, and lack of routine are some of the other factors responsible for respiratory difficulties.

Ayurvedic Remedies

The lungs are vital organs of the body that support the respiration and circulation process, functioning 24/7 effectively for us to live healthily. A wrong diet, inhalation of harmful toxins, and pollution develop many disorders in the respiratory system. Ayurvedic guidelines are quite helpful to cure many respiratory diseases as well as maintain a healthier system.

Here are some of the herbal remedies that can help to strengthen the respiratory system and to relieve the symptoms:

Vasak (*Adhatoda vasica*)

Vasak has long been used in ayurvedic medicine for soothing sore throat, common colds, respiratory infections, cough, acute bronchitis, chronic bronchitis, asthma, and breathing difficulties. Vasak leaves are commonly used as a home remedy for helping children sleep in cases of excessive nighttime coughing. Vasicine and vasicinone bioactive compounds present in the Vasak leaves possess potent antitussive and expectorant properties, which help to thin the mucus and expel it out of the body. This clears the respiratory tract and eases breathing. Vasak can help with both vata- and kapha-induced respiratory disorders.

Holy basil

Holy basil is a popular household herb found in every Indian home. For centuries, basil leaves have been used as a standalone treatment for all kinds of respiratory difficulties and common ailments. Its expectorant and antitussive properties are well-researched. Eugenol is the active principle of basil that has been shown to possess antibacterial, antiviral, anti-inflammatory, antifungal, and analgesic abilities, which altogether help in treating upper respiratory tract infections. The anti-inflammatory and analgesic abilities also help in soothing inflammation of respiratory pathways and ease breathing. Basil is also a great immune booster and supports natural healing.

While basil leaves are extremely potent in themselves, they make an even more powerful combination with honey and ginger. A decoction made by boiling basil leaves and mixed with honey and some warming spices like ginger, cinnamon, cloves, and cardamom is a popular home remedy for sinus blockages, cough, cold, viral infections, and breathing problems. This drink can also be taken as an herbal supplement for boosting general immunity.

Black pepper

The pungent, hot, sharp qualities of black pepper make it an extremely potent medicine against any kind of kapha disorder. It is a powerful expectorant that works almost instantly. Its warming effect helps in thinning the mucus and encourages their drainage. Piperine compound present in black pepper is known to have a strong antimicrobial effect that alleviates symptoms of common cold, cough, sore throat, and bacterial and viral infections.

Furthermore, black pepper can enhance the body's adaptability against environmental stressors, therefore enhancing the immunity against allergies caused by pollutants. As a stimulating pungent spice, black pepper is also perfect for enhancing the digestive agni, which helps prevent mucus accumulation and reduces the risk of respiratory disorders.

Astragalus

It is an incredible herb for strengthening and lubricating the lungs' capacity and to treat disorders like common cold, cough, flu, respiratory infections in the respiratory tract, and allergies.

Pippali

Pippali is an excellent ayurvedic herb that supports lung function, releasing mucus and sinus congestion. As per traditional preparation, boil ten pieces of pippali in milk and drink to release mucus and to cure a common cold, cough, bronchitis.

Ginger and garlic cloves

The anti-inflammatory properties of ginger are effective to fight with the root cause of the problems related to the respiratory tract. Two teaspoons of ginger juice mixed with two crushed garlic cloves may prove effective to release the accumulated mucus from the airways.

Bay leaf + pippali + honey

A mix of one-half teaspoon of ground bay leaf + one-quarter teaspoon of pippali + one teaspoon of honey is good to prevent chronic symptoms of asthma. As per expert advice, the patient can take two to three times a day.

Turmeric + neem (*Azadirachta indica*) + guggul

A mix of these herbs is good to fight any kind of allergies, loss of appetite, and diseases of the lungs.

Panchakarma for Asthma treatment

There are various respiratory disorders in which asthma is the most important. There are different types of asthma. Ayurveda and yoga therapy can be combined to treat and cure asthma. Panchakarma, herbal medicines, and ayurvedic diet are the main methods to treat asthma.

The main panchakarma therapies applied for asthma treatment are vaman, virechana, and nasya.

Vaman is one of the five therapies of panchakarma, which is therapeutic vomiting or medicated emesis. Vaman is done to remove toxins, especially from the respiratory and gastrointestinal tracts.

Virechana is a purification therapy that can prevent and heal several physical, mental, and emotional disorders. This therapy is for treating diseases that emerge from the vitiation of pitta dosha. By applying for the ayurvedic medicines, toxins are expelled via the anal route and is an important therapy in curing asthma.

Nasya includes the application of herbal oils, powders, or juices through the nasal route. It is best for disorders of the throat, nose, and ear. Nasya mainly purifies the nasal passage.

Vasti is an important panchakarma practice for balancing vata-related disorders. It promotes the elimination of excess vata dosha through the anus in the form of an enema.

Herbal Medicines and Ayurvedic Diet for Asthma Treatment

Always consume a glass of warm milk mixed with turmeric every night. This helps to fight cold infection and lung diseases. Ginger juice has anti-inflammatory properties, which can help to get rid of pollutants from the lungs.

Consume fresh ash gourd, honey, and lemon juice mixture or separately each one to bring lots of positive prana to the body and the mind system. Avoid onion and garlic, which are highly negative pranic food and can harm the pranic flow. Orange, lemon, carrots, etc., are good for lung infections as they are rich in vitamin C.

Always eat hot and warm food soon after cooking. Cold and rotten food consumption leads to respiratory infections. Consumption of cold water and cold dairy products should be avoided to keep the respiratory system healthy.

Yoga Therapy for Respiratory Disorders

Yoga therapy for respiratory disorders includes all breathing exercises and warm-up exercises, surya namaskar, most of the forward-bending, backward-bending, and twisting yogasanas, and all types of pranayamas.

Yoga breathing exercises are powerful practices to expand lung capacity and eliminate any breathing difficulties if regularly practiced. Yogasana, like bhujangasana, pavanamuktasana, ardha kati chakrasana, padahastasana, paschimottanasana , janushirshasana, sarvangasana, and ardha matsyasana, is a practice that is highly beneficial to cure asthma and other breathing difficulties.

The practice of surya namaskar for thirteen rounds followed by ten minutes of savasana can bring increased lung capacity and high breathing efficiency and also a balanced function of ida and pingala nadis.

Kapalbhati pranayama, bhastrika pranayama, and nadi shuddhi pranayama are the most beneficial pranayama practices to cure asthma and other breathing disorders. Similarly ujjayi and bhramari pranayamas are also beneficial to rejuvenate the breathing and lung capacities.

Yogic processes, from cleansing processes to savasana, purify the body and mind of the patient and help to cure respiratory disorders. The patient needs to follow step-by-step yogic treatment processes not only to strengthen the functional capacity of the lungs, but to also multiply the immune power to fight with allergies.

Yogic Kriyas (Cleansing Processes)

Jala neti

The ancient yoga system explains that jala neti brings miraculous solutions to various respiratory problems such as asthma, bronchitis, chronic sinus, migraine, sleep disorder, seasonal cold & cough, and allergies. The regular practice of jala neti increases the resistance capacity of the respiratory mucosa and functional capacity of the alveoli.

- Prepare salt water by adding half a teaspoon of salt to a neti pot of warm water.
- Stand with legs apart.
- If you start with the right side first, tilt your head gently to the left and insert the spout of the pot into right the nostril.
- Then open your mouth slightly (Breathing must be done with your mouth open throughout the process) and adjust the tilt of your head up to a point where the water starts flowing from your right nostril to the left nostril. Let it flow slowly till the pot is empty.
- Repeat on the other side.
- Once completed, close your ears with your thumbs and blow out forcefully through your nostrils the excess water in order to clear the nasal passages.

Asanas (Yoga Poses)

A healthier respiratory system is essential to avoid and to cope up with chronic diseases like asthma and COPD. Various yogic practices are highly effective to strengthen the respiratory system. Respiration is vital for every living being and affects all other functions of our body. Guided practice of yoga asanas, breath control, and regulation techniques are extremely useful for improving the breathing efficiency and decreasing inflammation.

- **Surya namaskar (sun salutation)**

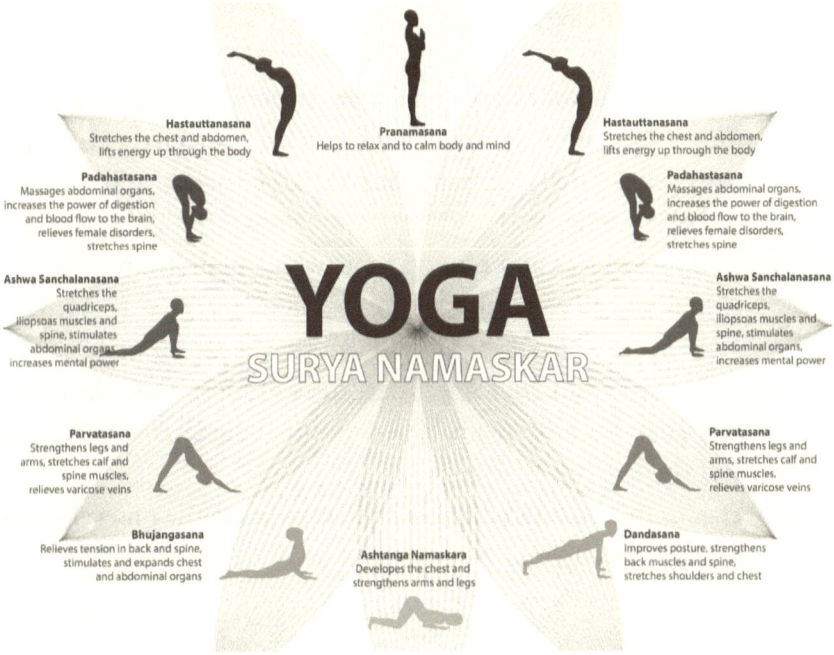

It comes as a complete package to stimulate and strengthen the overall body system and bonus to the respiratory system. The twelve successive asanas with a proper breathing technique are helpful to strengthen and to open up the lungs, air sacs, bronchioles, trachea, and nerves of the respiratory system.

- **Savasana (corpse pose)**

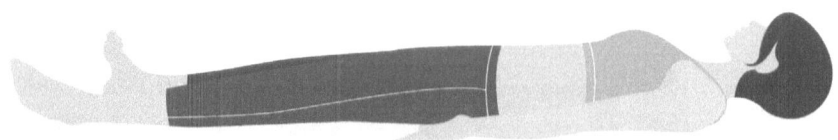

After sun salutation, savasana allows the body to absorb and integrate the energy generated during the practice into the muscle memory, mind, and nervous system. It is helpful to reduce stress and pain due to pulmonology.

- Lie down on your back. Feet apart, arms alongside your body, turn your palms upward facing toward the ceiling. Collapse your whole body, soften your facial muscles, and make a beautiful smile.
- Close your eyes and observe your whole body from your toes all the way up to head.
- Now, at each inhalation and exhalation, relax your body part by part. Start from your lower part (toes to hips), then shift your awareness to the upper part (from your abdomen to your neck), and finally your head region.
- Stay in this position for about ten minutes while observing the changes throughout your body.

- **Setu bandhasana (bridge pose)**

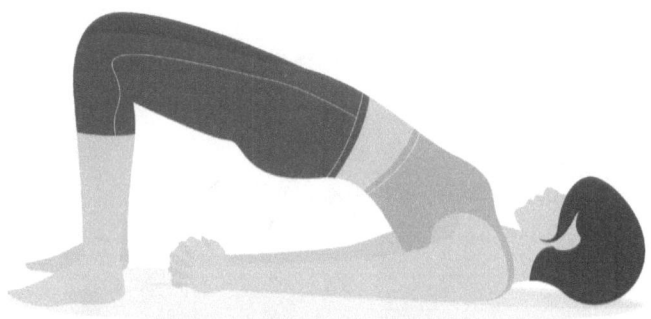

This asana also known as ardha sarvangasana (half-shoulder stand) is a useful pose for regulating the breathing process and strengthening the lungs. The pose opens up the chest muscles, and that helps the lungs to fill in more fresh air. This yogasana is beneficial for patients suffering from asthma, bronchiectasis, and high blood pressure.

- Lie down on your back, hands by the side of your body, and palms facing downward. Your feet should be hip-width apart.
- Bend your knees and bring your feet close to your buttocks. Ensure that your ankles and knees are in one straight line.
- Press your feet and while you inhale, lift your spine off the ground, vertebrae by vertebrae.
- Now, gently bend your shoulders and try to bring your chin to your chest.
- Let your shoulders, feet, and arms to support your weight.
- Maintain this pose for thirty to sixty seconds with slow inhalation and exhalation.
- Get your back down with deep exhalation and rest for a few seconds.
- Repeat for three to five times

- **Matsyasana (fish pose)**

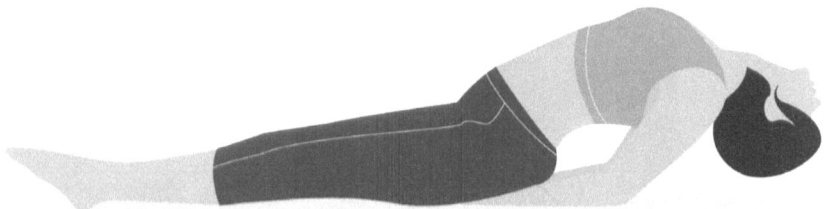

Matsyasana is an advanced asana that comes as a blessing for the respiratory system. This pose increases inflow and outflow of oxygen to the lungs, increases the muscle capacity, and helps to fight respiratory disorders like asthma, bronchitis, etc.

- Lie down on your back, feet apart, and your arms by the side your body.
- Slide your hands, palms under your hips, and keep the palms facing the ground.
- Pressing into the elbows, use your arms to lift your chest up toward the ceiling, arching your spine, and gently resting the crown of the head on the ground with face and neck relaxed.
- Do not put any weight on the head.
- Stay in this position for about one minute with normal breathing.
- To release, slowly and gently lower the back of your head, neck, and then your spine back down to the ground. Bring out the hands from under the hips.

• **Bhujangasana (cobra pose)**

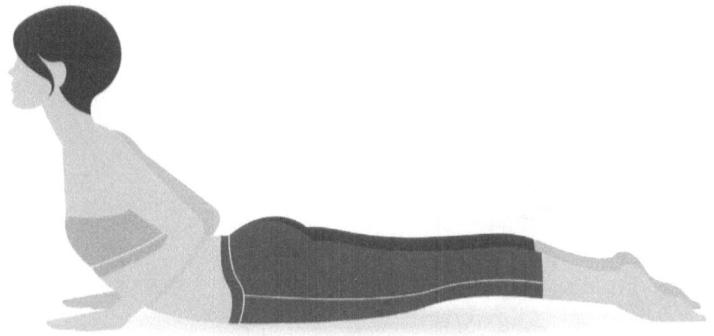

Bhujangasana relieves stress and fatigue with stretching and stimulating chest, lungs, shoulders, and abdomen. It opens the chest muscles and helps to improve the circulation of blood to pulmonary arteries and veins. Cobra pose is useful to control and manage many respiratory disorders as this pose gives good extension to the upper part of the spine, which is connected to lungs, rib cage, and windpipe.

– Lie down on your chest (in prone position), face down.
– Feet hip-width apart and the top of your feet flat on the floor with your toes spread out.
– Place your palms slightly lower than your shoulder, with the tips of your fingers right below your shoulder muscles and elbows close to your body pointing behind you and not outward.
– Inhale as you slowly lift your head and chest off the ground. Pull your shoulders back and your chest forward, but do not crunch your neck. Keep your shoulders away from your ears and bring your gaze up to the ceiling. Your arms bent at your elbows.
– Feel your stomach pressed on the ground and stay in this position with normal breathing for one minute.
– To release the pose, slowly bring your body down part until your forehead touches the ground. Then, place your hands under your head and rest your head on one side and breathe normally.

- **Ustrasana (camel pose)**

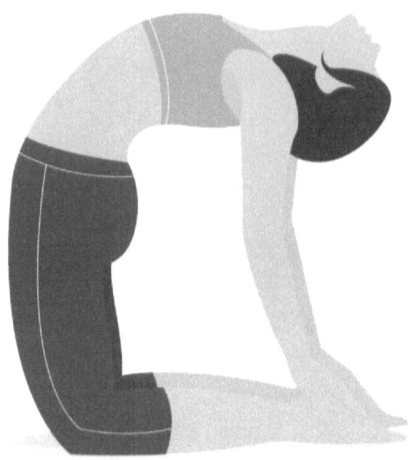

Ustrasana is a wonderful pose. It works to improve conditions of the digestive, respiratory, endocrine, and circulatory systems. Yoga experts recommend this asana for people suffering from asthma, bronchitis, thyroid, and spondylitis disorders.

- Sit on your heels, stretching your lower legs backward and keeping them together.
- Now, stand on your knees with your legs hip-width apart.
- Place your hands on your hips to support your back, fingers pointing forward, and your thumbs resting on your lower back facing toward each other. The elbows should be pointing behind.
- Keep your hips over your knees in one line.
- Now, as you inhale, round your shoulders back and open your chest. Then, with an exhalation, push your hips forward and slowly bend your spine backward from the waist.
- Once you feel stable, bring your palms down to the ankles of your feet one by one.

- Maintain this position for about a minute with normal breathing.
- To release, inhale and gently bring your hands on the lower back one by one.
- Simultaneously lift your head and chest up and come back to the initial position.
- You can rest in child pose or simply stretch your legs out straight in front of you (in dandasana) and relax.

- **Balasana (child pose)**

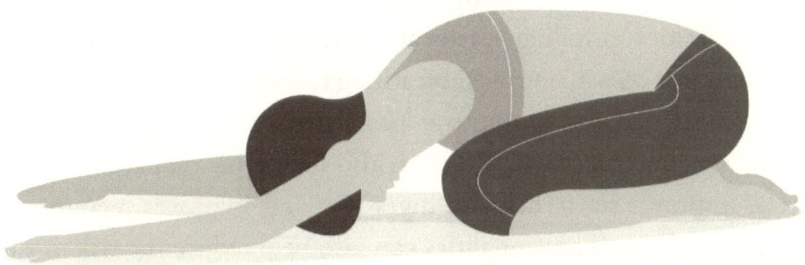

This relaxing pose improves the supply of blood to the brain and helps to alleviate fatigue, anxiety, and depression due to asthma attacks and COPD. Lower arm positions as well as compressing and squeezing the abdominal organs. Encourage the smooth flow of blood to the heart and complete exhalation. This condition improves the breathing pattern, which is especially beneficial for people suffering from asthma and chronic bronchitis.

- Sit on your heels and keep your knees hip-width apart.
- Then slowly inhale, and as you exhale, bring your chest down and rest it on your thighs.
- Stretch your arms forward in front of you.

- Relax and stay in this position while maintaining normal slow breathing for five minutes.
- Now, bring both hands by the side of your knees, press your palms, and slowly bring yourself up to the initial sitting position.

Pranayama

Vata is the energy responsible for breathing, and since it is also characterized by irregularity, any attempt to regulate breathing can help keep vata in balance. Pranayama, loosely translated as "control of the life force," is considered a powerful tool to enhance the well-being of respiratory organs. Prana (life force) is one of five sub-doshas of vata responsible for controlling heartbeat, inhalation, body-mind connection, and vitality of cells. Controlled breathing techniques used in pranayama practices are believed to improve lung capacity, clear out congestions, and relieve sinus blockages. Research also shows that pranayama reduces stress, improves sleep, helps in digestion, and improves memory and learning abilities. These qualities can also help reduce the risk of vata-induced respiratory disorders.

Yogic breathing techniques, which include calming, balancing, and stimulating , are the best practices for the respiratory system by improving and then strengthening the chest muscles. Pranayama are helpful for deep breathing, exchange of oxygen and carbon dioxide in the body, and to increase the flexibility of diaphragm which is the vital organ for respiratory function. According to recent studies, regular practice of pranayamas like bhastrika, anuloma-viloma, bhramari, and udgeeth are highly effective in improving lung function and to control disorders like chronic obstructive pulmonary disease (COPD), chronic bronchitis, emphysema, asthma, etc.

A patient with respiratory disorder needs to practice pranayama under the guidance of an expert to obtain the best benefits and to avoid negative consequences because of poor lung capacity.

Meditation

Meditation improves respiratory functions, cardiovascular parameters, and lipid profile, which extends the breath-holding capacity of the lungs. Though it is difficult, many studies explain that individuals with COPD or other forms of lung disease improve their sense of well-being and mood because of continuous meditation practice.

Naturopathic Therapy

The fundamental science behind naturopathic treatment is to increase the resistance capacity of the body to allergy, removing congestion of blood, better digestion, and accumulation of secretions, cleaning the morbid matters from the respiratory tract, better circulation, and improving the elasticity of the respiratory tissue. The following tips are helpful to control respiratory disorders:

- Take good care of your diet. Eat food that is easy to digest.
- Observe a day's fast every week in order to increase the efficiency of each and every cell of the body.
- Drink enough warm water with lemon juice during the fast.
- Perform enema or laghu shankha prakshalana (LSP) once a week to overcome constipation, which is another major cause for developing diseases like asthma.
- Avoid heavy meals, especially at night.
- Eat plenty of enzyme-rich foods (orange, papaya, guava, mango, rose apple), whole wheat flour, leafy vegetables, and boiled vegetables.
- Hot-water footbath in morning and evening is also helpful.
- Change your lifestyle. Living in healthy surroundings where there is plenty of clean air and sunlight helps the patient to restore the healthier respiratory system.

Conclusions

Respiratory diseases are progressive and life-threatening, which create conditions like breathlessness, pain, and inflammation to a patient. Globally, more than five hundred million cases are suffering from various respiratory disorders. As per hatha yoga philosophy, stress is the main cause of creating an imbalance in the lungs due to the adverse effect of our thought process and emotions. A healthy lifestyle, balanced diet, yoga practice, and meditation are helpful to reduce stress levels and to develop a strong immune system to fight against the cruel effects of chronic lung/heart diseases.

Chapter 7

Healing Spinal Disorders

The spine is composed of thirty-three individual bones called vertebrae, stacked one on top of another. The spinal cord passes through the spinal canal (a hole in the center of each vertebra). A combination of these stacks forms the vertebral column. The spine (vertebral column) is divided into four sections:

Cervical (C): (nape–topmost part)
Thoracic (T): (chest–middle part)
Lumbar (L): (lower back–lower part)
Sacral (S): (pelvis and tailbone–in-between hips)

The backbone/spine, which is made up of thirty-three separate vertebrae and supports to carry the weight of the entire body, is an immensely significant organ of the human body. The spinal cord is the main pathway for the transmission of information between the brain and rest of the body and is one the most important parts of every living being. The spinal cord is protected by bones, discs, ligaments, and muscles.

Spinal cord disorders are a major medical (neurologic) and financial problem because of their high prevalence. Spinal disease refers to a variety of backbone impairment conditions caused by a variety of factors, including old age, degenerative changes, spinal cord injury, accidents, infections, tumors, bone changes, or other medical conditions. Degenerative conditions that come with old age like arthritis, chronic back pain, difficulty in movement, and weakness are the most common spinal disorders. There are a number of spinal cord disorders that may originate outside the cord or inside the cord. The following are few common spinal disorders:

Deformities by birth

These include different sizes and shapes of the vertebrae and misaligned joints. Though surgery comes in the first place to overcome these issues, yoga plays a vital role to control after surgery complications as well as to cure minor deformities.

Accidents

Most of the time, accidents cause severe trouble to damage the vertebrae and injury to the disc. According to different medical reports, spinal disorders are important health problems, imposing an enormous financial burden upon the individual as well as the health care system, mainly due to road traffic accidents.

Compression of the spinal cord

Compression means unwanted pressure on the spinal cord. The spinal cord may be compressed by bone (which may arise because of cervical spondylosis, narrowing of the spinal canal, or a fracture).

Arthritis and bone spurs

Osteoarthritis causes severe joint inflammation and pain due to the breakdown of the cartilage of the joints and discs in the nape and lumbar region. Sometimes, the extra bone that may grow on joints, compresses the spinal cord or nerve roots, and develops weakness and pain in the arms or legs.

Blockage of the blood supply

The blockage of blood supply to arteries not only creates problems with the spinal cord, but also develops a big problem for the brain, as vertebral and internal carotid arteries supply blood to the brain. Blood clots and atherosclerosis are the major causes of blockage of blood supply to the arteries carrying blood to the spinal cord.

Holistic therapies available in yoga and ayurveda are sought as safe and effective treatments for long-term management of many of these conditions.

While any of the three doshas can cause spinal diseases, degenerative disorders are mostly a result of excess vata accumulation. Genetic factors, diet, and lifestyle changes may also play a role in developing these conditions in old age. With the natural aging process, oxidative stress and inflammation of cells can cause several degenerative changes in the body. Osteoarthritis, rheumatoid arthritis, and chronic back pain are some of the changes caused by the natural wear and tear of aging. Infections or injuries can further accelerate the natural breakdown of cartilage tissues, worsening these symptoms.

In the long run, spinal cord disorders may develop serious problems such as full loss of spinal movements, neurological problems, weak bladder functions, bedsores, etc. Many ayurvedic herbs and panchakarma procedures have been in use to treat such worst conditions for a long time.

Ayurvedic Therapy for Spinal Disorders

Ayurveda identifies that all spinal disorders are the result of vitiated vata and weakness of bones and muscles. Lower back pain, lumbar spondylitis/spondylosis, cervical spondylitis, lumbar or spinal stenosis, slip disc or herniated disc, sciatica, etc., are common spinal disorders. Most of the problems and treatments of neurological disorders and spinal disorders are closely related as the spine is the center of the nervous system, and all the muscles and the nervous system are mutually associated. The nervous system is made up of two major divisions: the central nervous system (consisting of the brain and spinal cord) and the peripheral nervous system (consisting of all other neural elements).

Generally, panchakarma, including abhyanga (body massage) padabhyanga (feet massage), kizhi (pinda sweda), ayurvedic medicines, and ayurvedic diet are integrated to treat all types of spinal disorders. Kizhi (pinda sweda) is usually recommended for the aching joints and muscles commonly associated with arthritic conditions, back pain, and muscle stiffness. Pinda sweda or kizhis are cotton boluses with a mixture of many herbs in podikizhi massage, which is of twelve herbs dipped in medicated oils. It is effective in treating neuromuscular diseases like many of the spinal disorders, bringing back the natural body balance.

Lumbar stenosis is the narrowing of spaces of the lumbar spine, causing the morbidity in old age. Usually, surgical laminectomy is the only answer in conventional therapy. However, the disease can be better treated in ayurveda through panchakarma and ayurvedic rasayana treatment.

The treatment for cervical spondylosis is comprehensive and may include ayurveda internal medicines and external applications for mild cases and along with these, ayurveda panchakarma therapies in severe cases. Diet and lifestyle modifications are applied in both scenarios.

Lumbar spondylitis/spondylosis is treated with abhyanga (body massage), nadi swedana, and kativasti. The ayurvedic medicines used are trayodashanga guggulu, mahavata vidhama/vatagajankus rasa, and brihat vata chintamani rasa/ashwagandharishta.

Cervical spondylitis/spondylosis is treated with abhyanga, nadi swedana, and grivavasti. The main ayurvedic medicines used are trayodasanga guggulu, mahavata vidhama/vatagajankus rasa, brihat vata chintamani rasa, dalmularista, or ashwangandharishta.

Sciatica syndrome is treated with abhyanga, nadi swedana, and kativasti. Ayurvedic medicines used are trayodasanga guggulu, mahavata vidhama or vatagajankus rasa, ekangavir or khajankari rasa, brihat vatachintamoni rasa, balarista or ashwagandharishta.

Ankylosing spondylitis is treated with shali pinda sweda. Ayurvedic medicines used are trayodasanga guggulu, maha yogaraj guggulu, mahavata vidhama rasa, maha rasnadi kwath, or dasamularista or ashwagandharista.

Lower back pain is always treated with pinda sweda (kizhi) or podikizhi (podi pinda sweda). Ayurvedic medicines used are ashwagandharista or balarista or vatankusa rasa.

Panchakarma Therapy

Panchakarma is a series of five therapies designed to detoxify the body inside-out. This intensive treatment is considered ideal for middle-age people. It is believed that these therapies restore the body's natural balance and rejuvenate tissues. Panchakarma is a deep-tissue purification program that seeks to undo the damage of aging, wrong eating and lifestyle practices, genetic predispositions, hormonal imbalances, and wear and tear of important bodily tissues.

Panchakarma therapies are believed to cleanse all the organs of toxins left out by diseases, restore dosha imbalance, clear out metabolic waste from neuromuscular junctions, improve digestion, enhance nutrient absorption, and boost immunity against diseases. However, the primary aim of panchakarma is to improve longevity and rejuvenate tissues. Ayurveda recommends these therapies for many degenerative disorders, including spinal problems and neurological disorders.

Oil Massage Therapy

Self-massage with nourishing oils is the easiest way to practice self-care. Ayurveda recommends self-massage every day for everyone, regardless of age. In fact, oils are given such a special place in ayurveda that in Sanskrit, oil is synonymous with love. Ayurveda believes that oil massage makes one feel the same way as receiving love!

Oils are believed to have a grounding effect on the light, dry, rough, moving qualities of vata. And since vata is responsible for most of the degenerative disorders, oil massage can help with many spinal disorders. Oils infused with soothing herbs are particularly effective as the anti-inflammatory effects of herbs help reduce inflammation of joints and relieve pain. In a 2017 trial conducted on sixty-four patients of spinal disorders, a two-week program of ayurvedic massage therapy significantly reduced chronic low back pain.

Yoga Therapy for Spinal Disorders

Though medical science treats many spinal disorders, it doesn't always bring the disease under control and many a time the patient encounters a number of side effects. When it comes to yogic treatment, yoga teaches the patient the technique to alleviate the pain as well as to cure the disorder without any side effects, and helps to lead as well as to maintain a healthy life.

Yoga therapies are well-recognized as an effective and sustainable approach to help with spinal disorders and back pain problems. A 2011 study using MR imaging techniques has shown that long-term yoga practitioners are at a lower risk of developing degenerative disc disease.

If anyone practices yoga systematically and in the right way daily, one will never get any back pain or spinal problems in their lifetime. Also, if the proper practice of yoga is performed daily, one can cure any type of spinal disorder within a period of two to three months.

Yoga not only means practice in a yoga center, but it also means how you sleep, how you walk, how you sit, and how you work. Since all spinal disorders are lifestyle disorders, the correct way to treat them is to correct the lifestyle.

Most of the spinal problems originate due to the wrong way of sleeping. So, if you sleep keeping your head toward east, west, or south (and never toward north), the direction of the mind will be peaceful and healthy. Also, sleep on your right side with your legs forward by bending your legs at the knees and sleep like that throughout the night. One never gets back pain or one can cure any back pain by sleeping in this manner. This is lifestyle correction for back pain problems. Follow it.

Yoga breathing exercises, warm-up exercises, loosening, rotating exercises, and all types of yoga asanas and surya namaskar are highly beneficial to cure all spinal disorders. One has to do with slow and little care when the pain is severe at the neck or back.

Pranayama, especially vibhaga pranayama (sectional breathing), nadi shuddhi pranayama, ujjayi pranayama, and bhramari pranayama followed by fifteen to thirty minutes of meditation can also help to detoxify and rejuvenate the nervous system associated with the spine and reduce the mental rigidity or mental stiffness to ease your mind, thereby the mind and body are very relaxed. Also, pranayama increases pranic flow in the spine and nervous system, helps to reduce the neuro spinal pain, and improves the neurophysiological functions to cure internally within a period of two to three months.

Yoga Asanas (for first two to three months)

- **Savasana (corpse pose)**

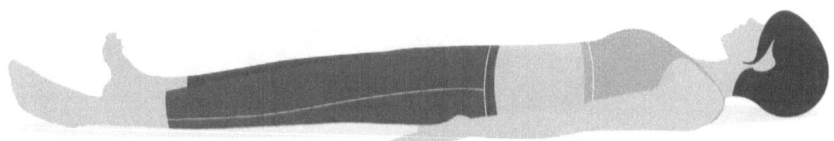

A patient of faulty spinal condition goes with lots of mental and physical pain. Five to ten minutes of savasana helps to reduce the pain and to start an effective session.

- Lie down on your back. Feet apart, arms alongside your body, turn your palms upward facing toward the ceiling. Collapse your whole body, soften your facial muscles, and make a beautiful smile.
- Close your eyes and observe your whole body from your toes all the way up to head.
- Now, at each inhalation and exhalation, relax your body, part by part. Start from your lower part (toes to hips), then shift your awareness to the upper part (from your abdomen to your neck), and finally your head region.

– Stay in this position for about ten minutes while observing the changes throughout your body.

• **Dandasana (staff pose)**

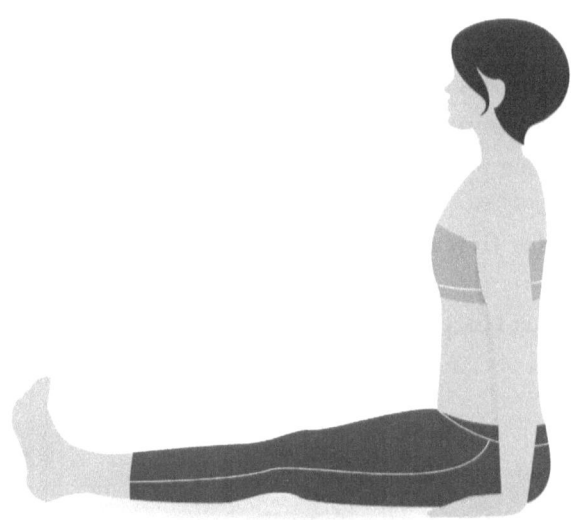

Regular practice of this exercise for one to two months will increase the muscle strength and alleviates pain due to sodalities.

– Sit comfortably on the ground with your spine erect and your legs stretched out in front of you.
– Press your buttocks on the ground and align your head to straighten and lengthen your spine.
– Keep your legs parallel to each other, press your heels, and flex your feet. Your toes should be pointing upward.
– Place your palms by the side of your hips on the ground to support your spine. Your torso straight and shoulders relaxed.
– Breathe normally and stay in this position with your legs relaxed for about one minute.

- **Vajrasana**

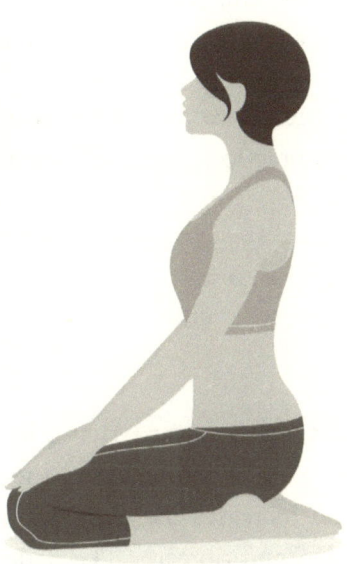

Every patient of spinal disorder needs to practice vajrasana as the initial position. Place your forehands beside the knees. Press the waist below and hold the neck backward. Your hands need to sustain the body weight. The patient needs to take great care while practicing this asana, because of the stimulation in the spinal cord.

- Kneel down and keep your lower legs together. Try to bring your big toes and heels as close as possible. If you have stiff ankles, roll a towel underneath to support the joint and arch of ankles.
- Gently rest your buttocks, your heels, and your thighs on your calf muscles.
- Then place your hands on your knees and set your gaze forward. Keep your head straight.
- Now, focus on your breath and observe your breathing pattern, how you inhale and exhale.

- You may close your eyes for good concentration of your breathing and to calm your mind.
- Stay in this position for at least five to ten minutes.

After practicing the above asanas for two to three months, the patient can follow the practices given below under the guidance of an experienced therapist.

Cleansing Practices

Uddiyana bandha

Uddiyana bandha, "the upward flying lock," is a good help to stretch and stimulate ganglia connected to the vertebra. This bandha pulls in the belly and increases the elasticity of nerves connected to the spine, core muscles, and rib cage. The patient should practice this bandha at a later stage under the supervision of an expert.

- In standing position, keep your feet hip-width apart. Bend your knees and lean slightly forward.
- Now, place your hands on your thighs and keep your arms straight.
- Take a few breaths and let your body relax.
- Exhale completely and hold your breath.
- Now, holding your breath, suck your navel in, all the way back to your spine. Then slowly lift it up toward your rib cage.
- Hold it for as long as you feel comfortable.
- To release, as you inhale, let go the abdominal muscles without gasping and return to standing position.
- Rest for a while and repeat the same practice for another five times.

The best time to practice uddiyana bandha is early in the morning, with empty stomach and bowels. It's *not* advisable for individuals with high blood pressure, hernia, ulcer, during pregnancy, and menstruation.

Asanas (Yoga Poses)

- **Tadasana (mountain pose)**

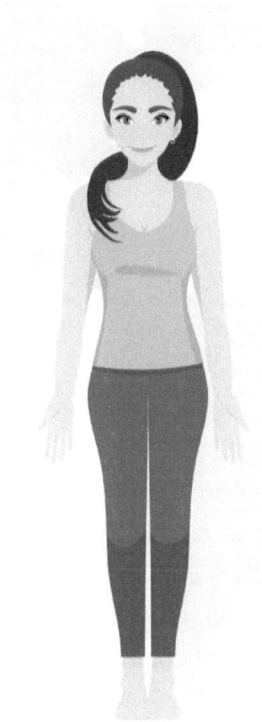

It is a basic and fundamental standing asana that pulls the tailbone downward and pushes toward the chest, thus increasing the weight-bearing capacity of the spine. Tadasana improves posture and comes in the first position to get relief from back pain.

- Stand straight, with heels slightly apart and toes touching each other.
- Pull up your kneecap to help engage your thighs.
- Arms by the side of your body with your palms facing forward and fingers widely spread.
- Lift up and widen your chest. Draw your shoulders back and relax.

- Lift the crown of your head up to elongate your neck.
- Gaze forward with your face relaxed.

- **Katichakrasana (standing spinal twist)**

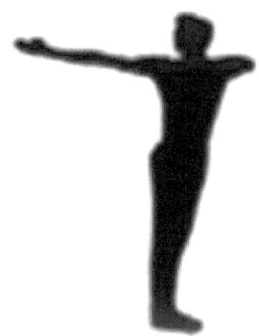

It is a waist-rotating standing yoga pose, which is good to develop the flexibility of the nerves connected to the spine and effective for spinal injuries and disorders. It is a great help to contract and expand the muscles of the neck, back, and love handles, and gives a calming massage to the entire vertebral column.

- Stand straight with your feet together and arms by the side of your body.
- As you inhale, stretch your hands forward at shoulder level with your palms facing each other and parallel to the ground (palms should be shoulder-width apart).
- Exhale and gently twist from the waist to the right and look back at your right shoulder.
- Maintain this position with slow breathing for one minute.
- Inhale and come back to center.
- Exhale and gently twist from the waist to the left and look back at your left shoulder.
- Maintain this position with slow breathing for one minute.
- Inhale and come back to center.
- Repeat this practice few times on both sides.

- **Pawanmuktasana (wind relieving)**

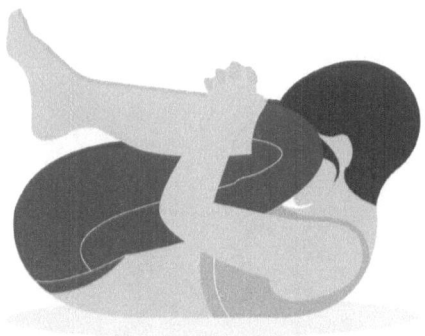

The wind-relieving pose is a supine warm-up exercise for the spine. Regular practice of this asana is helpful to control and manage conditions like scoliosis, lordosis, and kyphosis.

- Lie down on your back with your feet together and arms by the side of your body.
- Inhale, and as you exhale, draw both knees toward your chest and press your thighs against your abdomen with clasped hands.
- Inhale again, and as you exhale, lift your head and chest off the ground and place your chin on your knees.
- Stay in this position for as long as possible with deep, long breaths, in and out.
- Inhale, and as you exhale, slowly lower down your legs on the ground and rest in supine position for a few seconds.
- Repeat the same practice for another 3 to 5 rounds.

- **Anantasana (side-reclining leg raise)**

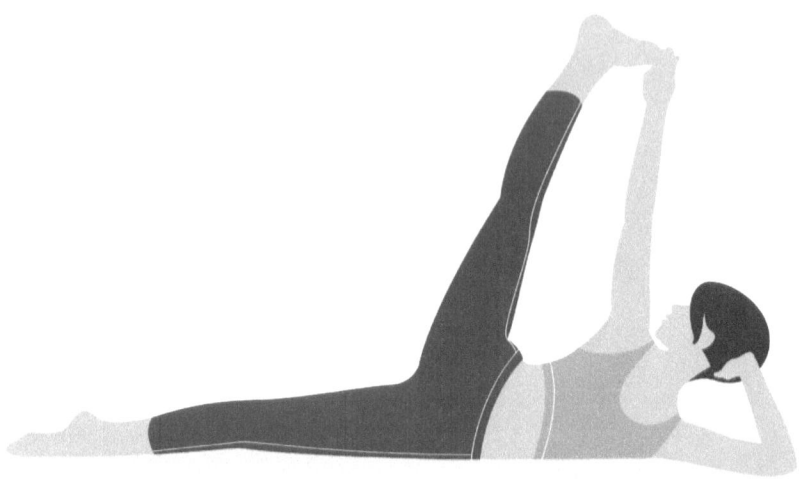

It is a simple asana and easy to practice. It opens the hip flexors, hamstrings, and groins, and reduces lower back pain by stimulating the lower section of the spine.

- Lie down on the right side with the left foot over the right. Press your right heel on the ground and maintain the balance using your foot.
- Rest your head on your right hand.
- Bend your left knee and draw it toward your chest. Then use your left hand to grab your big toe.
- Slowly pull your left leg up toward the ceiling and keep it above your left shoulder. Make sure that the sole of your left foot is facing upward to the ceiling.
- Stay in this position for one minute with normal breathing.
- Now, bring your left leg down and rest for a few seconds in supine position.
- Do the same on the other side.

– Repeat the same practice for both sides for another 3 to 5 rounds.

• **Shalabhasana (locust pose)**

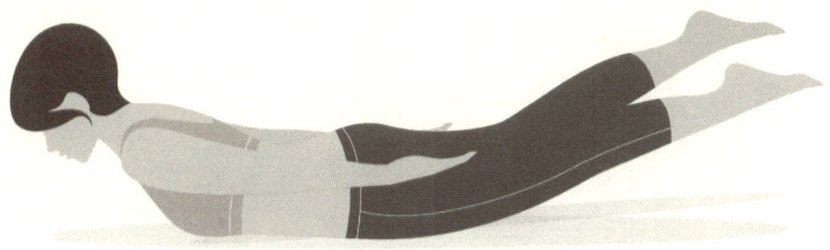

The locust pose helps to treat problems with the spine by compressing the entire vertebral column. This pose helps to provide relief from backache, sciatica, and slipped disc.

– Lie down in prone position with your abdomen/tummy on the floor.
– Make a fist with your hands and slide it under your thighs with the back of your hands on the ground. Keep your body relaxed.
– As you inhale, slowly lift both legs upward as high as you can without bending your knees.
– Stay in this position for one minute with normal breathing.
– To release, at exhalation, slowly bring your feet down.
– Then turn your back and rest in savasana (corpse pose) for a few minutes.

- **Bhujangasana (cobra pose)**

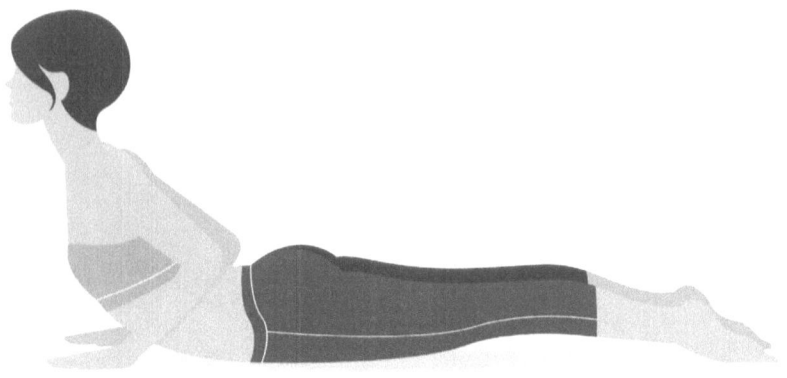

It is an advanced pose that stimulates the entire spinal column. It increases the suppleness of the spine with abundance of blood supply to the nerves, rejuvenates the spinal cord, and tones the connecting muscles of the nape, shoulders, and lower back.

- Lie down on your chest (in prone position), face down.
- Feet hip-width apart and the top of your feet flat on the floor with your toes spread out.
- Place your palms slightly lower than your shoulder, with the tips of your fingers right below your shoulder muscles and elbows close to your body pointing behind you and not outward.
- Inhale as you slowly lift your head and chest off the ground. Pull your shoulders back and your chest forward, but do not crunch your neck. Keeping your shoulders away from your ears can bring your gaze up to the ceiling. Your arms bent at your elbows.
- Feel your stomach pressed on the ground and stay in this position with normal breathing for one minute.
- To release the pose, slowly bring your body down part, until your forehead touches the ground. Then, place your hands under your head, rest your head on one side, and breathe normally.

- **Marjariasana (cat pose)**

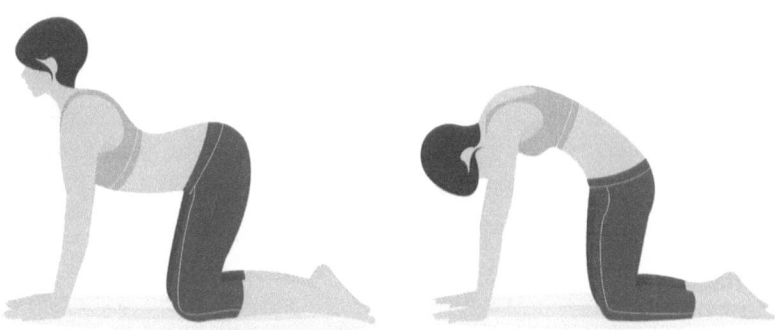

Marjariasana, also known as the cat pose, is a relaxing pose that relieves stress and tension of the spine and neck. It gives a gentle massage to the spinal cord as well as the vertebral column.

- Stand on all fours (your back will form a table top). Your knees and feet should be hip-width apart. Your shoulders and wrists in one line, and palms firmly on the ground with fingers widely opened.
- Gaze straight forward and keep your body relaxed.
- While i nhaling, lift your chin up and look up at the ceiling. Push your navel down and raise your tailbone up. Compress your buttocks.
- Stay in this pose for a few breaths.
- To release, while exhaling , curl in your shoulders , suck your belly in and drop your chin to your chest. Arch your back and relax your buttocks.
- Stay in this pose for a few breaths. This makes up one round.
- Repeat the movement and countermovement for five to 10 rounds.

Contraindications

A big *no* to all forward-bending asanas (The first and the foremost rule is, do not lean in a forward direction, because bending forward stretches the vertebrae nearer to each other and develops acute pain).

Avoid other asanas and pranayamas like sarvangasana, halasana, shirshasana (headstand), fast breathing, bhastrika pranayama, and any other pranayama with kumbhak (breath holding).

Pranayama

Millions of people face problems like lower back pain, neck pain, neck stiffness, and movement because of cervical spondylosis. The root cause of all these problems is insufficient nutrients and lack of flexibility of the spine. On the other hand, the regular practice of pranayama not only increases the flexibility of the spinal cord, but also provides an abundance of nutrients by increasing the flow of blood and oxygen to the nerves connected to the spine.

Anulom vilom (belly breathing) and bhramari pranayamas are quite helpful in activating the degenerative spine as well as to strengthen the nerve ganglia. A patient of spinal disorder must practice under the supervision of the healer/expert to obtain the best benefit out of it.

Meditation

Meditation is an excellent therapy to control and manage problems with the brain and spinal cord (nervous system). Research shows that ten to twenty minutes of mindfulness meditation on the navel center is effective in treating spinal disorders as the patient reduces stress, regains weight wearing capacity of the spine, and peaceful sleep.

Naturopathic Therapy

Naturopathy lays emphasis on the right diet and regular exercise to control these disorders. A healthy diet rich in calcium and protein like lots fresh fruits and green leafy vegetables. Milk is essential for the patient of such conditions.

- Drink juice of giloy with an empty stomach in the morning.
- Eat salad—plenty of green vegetables, beetroot, and carrot.
- A mix of turmeric and shilajit in milk can be effective.
- Stretch your hands above the head every time you get up from your sitting or sleeping position.
- Regular exercise is needed to strengthen your muscles, for a healthy weight is key to avoid as well as to control many vertebral problems.

Conclusions

"Every year, around the world, nearly five hundred thousand people suffer a spinal cord injury. The majority of spinal cord injuries are due to road traffic crashes, falls, or violence." (WHO)

A healthy lifestyle has the biggest influence on back pain and spinal disorders. Every patient needs to develop healthy habits such as a good diet, exercising, stretching, yoga, and meditation to overcome many health disorders developed due to spinal injury.

Chapter 8

The Purpose and Importance of Breathing and Relaxation in Yoga

The definition of yoga is "that which unites." That means it is the science of attaining union of our jeevatma (individual soul) with the paramathma (supreme soul).

To reach that level, one may take a long way of practice, which Patanjali Maharshi explained in his classical text, *Yoga Sutras Ashtanga Yoga* (The Path of Eight Limbs/Steps). If one takes the path of this yoga, one can reach the ultimate union with the supreme soul.

These eight steps are yama, niyama, yogasana, pranayama, pratyahara, dharana, dhyana, and samadhi. Both yama (social disciplines) and niyama (self-disciplines) are ethical and moral practices.

Even though the ultimate union takes place in the higher level of yoga, the initial level of the union takes place between the body and mind, which are united by the process of conscious breathing or breathing with awareness.

Chapter 9

The Three Pillars of Yogasana Practice and Its Benefits

Yogasana practice always starts with breathing, loosening (joints), and warm-up exercises. So the first thing one learns in yoga is how to breathe properly, systematically, and scientifically. These yoga breathing and warm-up exercises will help the new yoga practitioner to enhance his breathing capacity, expand his lung capacity, and coordinate and rejuvenate all the body and mind system. After a week of breathing and warm-up practices, one is ready to practice yogasana.

Yogasana practice focuses on three pillars, which are breathing, relaxation, and awareness. Breathing (movement of prana, the life force) should be done consciously or with awareness. In yoga, breathing is used as a tool to connect the body, mind, and consciousness by deepening awareness.

In yogasana, the main focus of the practitioner should be on breathing, relaxation, and awareness to get the real benefit from the practice. Breathing consciously while in any yoga pose connects the mind with the body and the self-consciousness, which deepens the awareness. Noting the physical movements, the posture itself, breath control, synchronization of breath with body movements, mental counting, sensations in the body, movements of prana, concentration on an area of the body or chakra, and more precisely, any thoughts and feelings that may arise during the practice.

So the whole purpose of yoga is to be aware of every moment in your life. For that, we use breathing as an important tool or object. This perfects anyone to be present in this moment. What we call stress is nothing but unconscious living without focusing or awareness of these fundamental tools of life that are called breathing relaxation and awareness in every moment.

The practice of surya namaskar is a string of many yoga asanas that focuses on different postures, breathing or pranayama, and awareness followed by relaxation after the practice.

Relaxation in yoga is considered as the most vital practice. Warming up and cooling of the muscles are important in any exercise practice. Many yoga relaxation techniques are used to relax the body and mind. Savasana and yoga nidra are the two important relaxation techniques practiced in yoga. Savasana is practiced after each asana for one minute or less duration or a short duration of a maximum of ten minutes, while yoga nidra can go from thirty minutes to one-hour duration. Savasana or yoga nidra is practiced after performing all the yoga asana practice and after surya namaskar. Savasana practice is compulsory after surya namaskar.

The purposes of relaxation techniques like savasana and yoga nidra are:

- to cool down the body muscles
- to normalize our breathing patterns
- to relax our heartbeats
- to release body aches and tiredness
- to slow down and calm the mind
- to heal the body and mind by boosting immunity
- to release stress and tension from the body and mind
- to strengthen the nervous system and mind
- to energize the whole body system and mind
- to deepen the awareness and expand the consciousness

Yoga nidra can also give all the above results and apart from that, yoga nidra can eliminate deep-lying emotional stress and trauma, tension, and stress as it is a long duration practice of visualization and relaxation techniques. Research studies have shown that yoga nidra has the power to cure many mental and physical ailments like anxiety, depression, insomnia, and cancer.

Chapter 10

AUM (OM) Chanting and Benefits

Both savasana and yoga nidra practice includes the practice of chanting of A, U, M, and AUM (OM) as these sounds produce vibrations that have the power to make the body and mind relaxed and spiritual conscious awakened.

Chanting of "A" or akara chanting creates vibrations in the lower part of the body, below the navel. These vibrations enter into the cellular level, bringing vibrations to all parts of the muscles and nervous system. When the vibrations subside, relaxation deepens.

Chanting of "U" or U-kara brings the vibrations to the middle part of the body, thereby bringing vibration within the chest and abdominal region above the navel and below the chin. These vibrations stimulate the abdominal organs like the liver, stomach, pancreas, heart, and lungs. Hence, when the vibrations subside, it deepens the relaxation within these respiratory, circulatory, and digestive systems.

Chanting of "M" or M-kara brings vibrations to the upper part of the body, especially the head portion, above the chin. These vibrations stimulate the brain and other parts of the brain, like the hypothalamus, medulla, etc., thereby stimulating the thought process and mental functions. Hence, when these vibrations subside, the relaxation deepens within the brain and central nervous system, bringing calmness and peacefulness with the body and mind.

Finally, A, U, and M, when chanted together in one breath to feel the shifting of vibrations and realization of calmness manifesting in the three parts of the body, bring ultimate peacefulness to the body and mind.

Then, at the last, AUM-kara or OM chanting is practiced for awakening the consciousness within. As Patanjali says, OM-kara chanting introverts the mind and brings meditativeness or one-pointedness to the mind as the mind gets inverted toward the self with regular chanting of AUM (OM), which can lead anyone to meditation and samadhi in the higher states of practice.

OM-kara meditation is practiced by adopting the following mudras:

— A-kara chanting with chin mudra
— U-kara chanting with chinmaya mudra
— M-kara chanting with adi mudra
— A, U, M chanting together with brahma mudra

These mudras also awakened the lower, middle, and upper parts of the body while adopted.

During the practice of both savasana and yoga nidra, one should lie down like a corpse and should not move any part of the body while practicing, and the mind should be alert without sleeping to get all the benefits of the practice.

Chapter 11

Pranayama: The Science of Breathing and Its Benefits

Pranayama is the science of breathing. After mastering the posture (yogasana), one must practice the control of breathing or prana (pranayama) by stopping the motions of inhalation and exhalation.

Prana is the universal vital force that pervades the mineral world, vegetable kingdom, and animal kingdom including the human beings, where it manifests as pancha prana (five functions, as prana, apana, samana, vyana, and udana). Prana performs respiration, apana performs excretion, samana performs digestion, udhana performs speech, and vyana performs circulation of blood to the entire body.

Pranayama is the preparatory practice for dharana, a premeditated state, thereby reaching the state of meditation. When meditation perfects, the highest goal of samadhi or blissful state or union with the supreme soul will happen.

Hence, pranayama is a conscious breathing practice to reach the highest goal of yoga and life.

The breath may be stopped externally (bahya kubhaka, eternal breath retention), or internally (antar kumbhaka, internal breath retention) or checked in midmotion, and regulated according to place, time, and a fixed number of moments, so that the stoppage is either protracted or brief. Prana means life force and "ayama" means extension or stretching. Hence, by stretching the normal breath to a considerable time of length, one can control the vrittis (activities of mind), as Patanjali defined yoga as "Chitta vritti nirodhah."

In the classical textbook, *Hatha Yoga Pradipika* by Swami Swatma Rama, it says "Chale vate chittam chalet, nischalam vate nischalam bhavet," which means, when the breath moves, the mind moves, and when the breath stops, the mind stops. This shows the connection between our mind and breathing. Hence, by handling our breath, we can easily control our minds. By consciously slowing down the breath, we can slow down the wandering of the mind. This scientific observation by ancient yogis of India has become the foundation for the scientific method of breathing known as pranayama. This knowledge to understand the connection between breathing and the function of the mind also became the foundation for all yoga therapy techniques to treat the mind through pranayama, the breath control.

Bandhas are neuromuscular locks. In hatha yoga, three bandhas are applied. These are jalandhara bandha (chin lock), moola bandha (rectum lock), and uddiyana bandha (abdominal lock). When all three are applied, it's tri-bandha. They help in hatha yoga pranayama as safety valves. These are only applied to experienced yoga students.

By reducing the number of breaths per minute, hatha yogis can extend their lifespan. As you know, animals that breathe faster and more numbers per minute (twenty or more per minute) live a shorter life, like dogs and cats. While animals that breathe very slowly and breathe less breath per minute (less than six or eight per minute) live longer, like tortoises (150 years), crocodiles (300 years). By observing this, ancient hatha yogis found that, if one reduces the speed of breathing and breathe slowly and less the number of breaths per minute, they can extend their lifespan. This is how the method of pranayama came into practice.

The physical and mental benefits of pranayama practice are:

- Body and mind become calm and composed
- All the seventy-two thousand nadis are detoxified, especially by nadi shuddhi pranayama
- Complete detoxification of body and mind
- All nervous systems strengthened and nervous disorders will be cured

The spiritual benefits are:

- Body consciousness is reduced and self-consciousness is expanded
- The inner effulgence is uncovered
- The mind becomes capable of dharana (premeditative state)

There are more than nine pranayama techniques, which are useful breathing techniques in yoga to get physical, mental, spiritual benefits. These are as follows:

- **Sukha pranayama** - Easy breathing for learning the process of pranayama practice initially by watching different parts of the body where prana flows.
- **Kapalabhati pranayama** - For cleansing the frontal brain and lungs as the first preparatory detoxification process before starting daily pranayama. If you practice it slower, it is kapalabhati pranayama , and if you practice it faster, it is kapalabhati kriya.
- **Vibhaga pranayama** or **sectional breathing** - For preparing the lungs for full pranayama practice and to increase the lung capacity.
- **Bhastrika pranayama** - For heating the body to energize and get rid of laziness and lethargy. This can be useful in winter.

- **Seethali, seethkari,** and **sadantha pranayamas** - Cooling the body and stimulating the taste buds in the tongue and digestive system.
- **Chandra (left) anuloma-viloma** (anuloma = inhalation, viloma = exhalation) and **surya (right) anuloma-viloma** - For balancing the right and left sides of the body and its functions.
- **Chandra bhedana (intersect) pranayama** and **surya bhedana pranayama** - For balancing the left and right side of the body and its functions.
- **Nadi shuddhi pranayama** or **anula-viloma** or **nadi shodhana pranayama** - Forgetting spiritual awakening of consciousness within by getting rid of body consciousness. It balances the body, mind, and purification of seventy-two thousand nadis (nadi = prana energy flow channel).
- **Ujjayi pranayama** - For calming, soothing, and relaxing the mind, body, and nervous system. Good for all mental issues and well-being.
- **Brahmari pranayama:** For calming, soothing, and relaxing mental well-being.

Chapter 12

Meditation: Purpose, Benefits, and Types

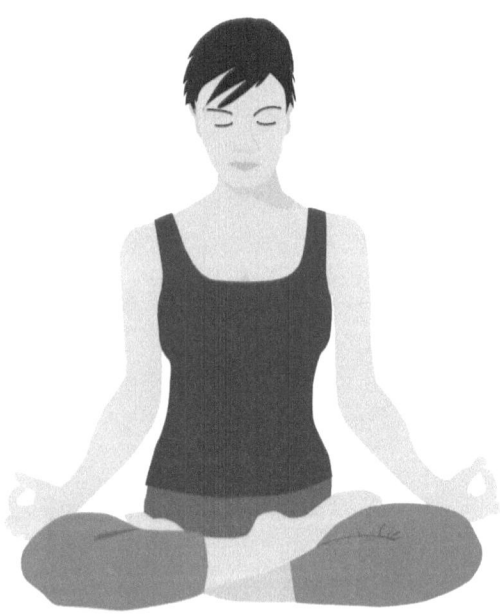

Dhyanam or meditation is the eighth step (limb) of Ashtanga yoga of Patanjali, as explained in his classical text, *Yoga Sutra*. The English word "meditation" does not completely derive the meaning of the Sanskrit word "dhyanam." In the state of dhyanam, there will be a continuous flow of concentration and effortless dwelling of mind toward a single object without any distractions.

On the other hand, the word "meditation" is used to describe some different uses of the mind, from contemplation and concentration to devotion and chanting. The word meditation might have derived from the same root as the Latin word "mederi," which means "to heal." Meditation can certainly be looked on as a healing process, emotionally, mentally, and also physically.

The meditative state is experienced as the highest state of existence. It is indispensable for spiritual life as breathing is for the process of living. Without meditation, one is like a blind man in a world of light, color, and joyfulness.

The Purpose of Meditation

The word yoga is derived from the Sanskrit word "yuj," which means "yoke" or merge. That means it is union. The union between the jeevatma (individual soul) with the paramathma (supreme soul). We are all individual souls who are separated from the supreme soul at the time of birth. That is why we all have that aspiration to reach that union with the supreme soul. This is why we are doing all kinds of small or big activities to reach that union one day. Meditation is considered as the easiest and the wisest way to reach that union.

So the ultimate purpose of yoga is union with the supreme self or God himself. This is the same purpose of meditation. Meditation is the highest method of yoga practice to achieve that union. Being the highest method, no one can start meditation at the beginning of the process. He has to start from the practice of yama and niyama, yogasana, pranayama, prathyahara, and dharana and then come to the state of meditation.

Patanjali, in his classical text *Yoga Sutra*, describes eight steps of Ashtanga yoga to reach the self-realization or union with the supreme self. These eight limbs of yoga practice is known as Ashtanga yoga or the yoga of eight limbs or eight steps. This yoga path in modern times is also known as raja yoga, as Swami Vivekananda called it.

The eight steps are:

- Yama (social disciplines)
- Niyama (self-disciplines)
- Asana (yogasana - physical posture)
- Pranayama (breathing technique for breath control)
- Prathyahara (sense control)
- Dharana (concentration)
- Dhyana (meditation)
- Samadhi (blissful state)

Samadhi or blissful state is the final stage or the result of the perfection of your meditation. Hence, meditation is a process, and the perfection of which can lead to liberation or moksha (salvation, according to Christianity), or self-realization (enlightenment), which is the only purpose of life and also the only purpose of meditation.

But in the modern times, people come to yoga and practice meditation as a process to heal their physical, mental, and emotional problems. So modern yoga practices are all aimed at getting physical and mental health benefits, which are usually the surficial benefits of yoga. No doubt meditation can cure all physical, mental, and spiritual health issues if practiced systematically and regularly with the help of a guru (enlightened master) or competent teacher. Meditation removes all the accumulated past karma, empties your karmic baggage, relieves you, lightens your burden of life, and makes you a new free soul.

In *Yoga Sutra*, yoga is defined by Patanjali as "Yogah chitta vritti nirodhah" (yogah = yoga, chitta = manas (mind stuff), vritti = activities, nirodhah = cessation). That means yoga is the process of stopping the activities of your mind. So when yoga achieves this goal of stopping the activities of mind, one realizes himself or reaches the state of samadhi. Because it is the mind that always takes you away from the true nature of your self.

Lord Krishna in *Bhagavad Gita* (B. G. 18–66) said, "Oh Arjun, if sleep and dreams disappear, you are your self." The simple meaning of this is that, when you can win your mind and its activities and be able to stop or still the mind, you will not get any sleep or dream and you become one with your self or get self-realized. That is the purpose of meditation.

According to the spiritual laws, a guru or enlightened master can only take the disciples to the highest paths of yoga, which are meditation and samadhi. One who meditates on his guru can easily reach the perfection of meditation, which is the state of samadhi, as explained by Lord Shiva in *Guru Gita*. Guru's physical form or formless nature (consciousness) is the source of meditation (Guru Gita).

According to Shirdi Sai Baba, an incarnation of Dattatreya Guru, as explained in his biography *Sai Satcharitra*, guru is necessary to reach the state of self-realization and that continuous practice of meditation is necessary. The simplest method that Shirdi Sai Baba recommends is to remember your guru all the time, and the dwelling mind upon guru's form, slowly get rid of the wandering nature, lose its fickleness, and merge with the guru's formless nature (consciousness). Hence, the self is the master or guru himself.

Benefits of Meditation

Meditation is considered as:

- an exercise for the expansion of consciousness and the exercise of deepening awareness
- a mental practice in which thinking and intuitive perceptions take place continuously
- a process of rejuvenating, rediscovering, enjoying, and using the positive qualities already latent within us
- a practice that can stabilize the emotions and attain a balance between the right and left brain functions, the balance of ida and pingala, thereby stimulating the function of sushumna nadi
- a practice that awakens the latent faculties of the mind and channels the thoughts toward mental, physical, and spiritual well-being
- a practice that channels the mind in a positive direction

- a practice that enables one to go beyond the five senses and achieve the non-individualistic nature
- safest practice to heal any physical, mental, and spiritual health problems and remove all impediments for spiritual growth

Spiritual benefits of meditation are:

- Peace of mind (shanti)
- Contentment (santhosha)
- Steadiness or stillness of body and mind (sthithi)
- Free from likes and dislikes (raga-dvesha)
- Free from ego (prakamya)
- Inner vision (divine drishti)
- Pure positive qualities (sattvic gunas)

Methods of Meditation

Meditation can be practiced in different ways. But the general rules are the same or similar. They are the following:

- Some people make an idea and follow it to arrive at a given result—this is an active meditation. If people want to solve a problem, they can meditate in this way even without knowing that they are meditating.
- Some people may sit down and try to concentrate on some object without following an idea—this can be concentrating on a point whether mental, vital, or physical, to intensify one's power of concentration.
- Some other people may sit down to arrive at true silence and tranquility. This is extremely difficult and it is nearly like taking bull by the horns.

Perception: The Mind as Our Instrument of Perception

In raja yoga (Ashtanga yoga), the mind is the instrument for looking inward and uncovering the inner self. The mind is a simple instrument through which the soul interacts with the world, including the physical body. This internal mental instrument is called the chitta in yoga. The chitta is often described as a lake, and in this mind-lake, waves of thought rise and fall away as a result of the impressions we take in from the external world. So sometimes the mind is restless and disturbed and sometimes it is calm, just like the surface of a lake. When the surface of the mind-lake is very disturbed, because many thoughts are rising like waves, we cannot see the bottom of the lake. We only glimpse the bottom when the waves have subsided and the lake is calm. Think of the bottom of the lake as the inner self, the spiritual center.

Types and Practices of Meditation

All of the meditation practices are done by sitting on a yoga mat or a piece of cloth spread on the floor. This is to avoid earthing of the body as the practice can make some energy changes in the physical and energetic level. After sitting in any comfortable posture or asana like sukhasana, swastikasana (crossed legs), siddhasana, vajrasana, ardha padmasana or padmasana, one can start the meditation. Hold chin mudra or prana mudra or any other suitable mudra for specific purposes. But generally, chin mudra is recommended for all, as chin mudra dissolves the ego and increases concentration.

The length of meditation depends on person to person. Ideally, fifteen minutes are recommended for beginners. A teacher can give guided meditation in the beginning. And after some time, one must practice himself. Swami Vivekananda said, start your meditation with a silent prayer to God and Mother Earth. In a regular yoga class, practice meditation after yogasana and pranayama.

Mindfulness meditation is a new term that people use for meditation that practices more awareness of whatever the mind does and being only the witness of all mental activities without stopping the thoughts. Almost all meditation is mindfulness in nature. There is no need to mention it separately. Pranayama meditation, transcendental meditation, and vipassana meditation are mindfulness meditation types.

The important types of meditation are:

1. **OM (AUM)-Kara Meditation**

OM (AUM) is a basic mantra and sacred syllable. It is the first sound of the universe or known as the pranava mantra or adi mantra (first mantra). It is the sound personification of Brahman or universal self. Patanjali, in *Yoga Sutra*, recommended practicing the chanting of OM repeatedly for a certain number of times regularly to take the mind inward-directed to the self. This will induce a meditative state for the mind, and practice of meditation after chanting of OM can slowly bring the calmness of mind and stillness of mind. This practice is done with simple chanting of OM for 9 or 15 rounds or 21 rounds or 27 or 54, or 108 times. Chanting OM for 108 times is always recommended. Then, after chanting for 108 times, sit for meditation for 15, 30, or 60 minutes with your mind focusing on the breath. This is OM-kara meditation.

Another variation of OM-kara chanting and meditation is nadanusandhana. It is OM-kara chanting with fine awareness. In this practice, OM is chanted as a combination of three sounds as A, U, and M. This can be chanted first separately and then together to bring vibrations of the lower, middle, and upper parts of the body. This kind of chanting and meditation is known as nadanusandana. This is very good for mental calmness and focus of mind to the inner self.

Practice

- Sit in any comfortable posture and hold chin mudra while chanting A-kara for five or nine times. First breathe in, and while breathing out, one has to produce the sound of Aa . . .
- Chant U-kara for five or nine times with chinmaya mudra in the middle of the thighs.
- Chant M-kara for five or nine times with adi mudra held at the base of the thighs.
- Chant all three together (A-U-M) for five or nine times with Brahma mudra held at both sides of the navel.

- After the end of the chanting, release the Brahma mudra and hold chin mudra and sit for meditation, mentally focusing on the breath, for fifteen, thirty, or sixty minutes. End the session with chanting of the prayer.

Benefits

- Chanting OM cures throat problems, voice problems, etc.
- Induces deep sleep and releases stress and tension
- The most effective benefit of this practice is calmness, stillness, and one-pointedness of the mind, suitable for long-time meditation.
- Nadanusandhana is a meditation technique for kids, mentally distracted people, and those who have excessive body pain (conducted in savasana).

2. **Pranayama Meditation**

In pranayama meditation, first, practice any pranayama for a certain number of cycles and then sit for meditation for some time. The most important pranayama for practicing meditation are nadi shuddhi pranayama, ujjayi pranayama, and brahmari pranayama. Hence, we can look at each one as different meditation practices as below:

a. Nadi Shuddhi (Anuloma-Viloma) Pranayama Meditation

Practice

- Sit in any comfortable posture, eyes closed with chin mudra in both hands.
- Watch your breath till your breath becomes normal.
- Then, take a full breath through both nostrils.
- Close the right nostril with your right thumb by holding the nasika mudra (vishnu mudra) and exhale through the left nostril.

- Then, again, inhale through the left nostril and close the left nostril with your right ring finger and exhale through the right nostril.
- Then, again, inhale through the right nostril. Then, close the right nostril with the right thumb and release through the left nostril. Now, one cycle of nadi shuddhi pranayama is completed.

Similarly, practice seven, nine, fifteen, or twenty-one cycles of nadi shuddhi pranayama.

- After the completion of the pranayama, release the nasika mudra and hold chin mudra on both hands.
- Sit for meditation with your mind focusing on the breath alone. Meditate for fifteen, thirty, or sixty minutes. Then, to close the session, chant the ending prayer and conclude the session.

Benefits

- This is the most effective pranayama meditation practice for spiritual progress as it can take away the body consciousness if practiced for a long period daily and regularly.
- Best for curing anxiety, depression, insomnia, and stress, as nadi shuddhi pranayama purifies seventy-two thousand nadis in our body.
- It can cure many physical, mental, and spiritual problems of life.

b. Ujjayi Pranayama Meditation (Ujjayi = Hissing Sound)

Practice

- Sit in any comfortable posture and adopt chin mudra or any mudra with your hands.
- While breathing, contract glottis in the throat and inhale deeply, as if you are breathing through your throat only.
- While exhaling, also contract the glottis in the throat, as if you are breathing through your throat only.

- The breathing should be slow, deep, and should be touching the upper palate while inhalation and exhalation, producing a hissing sound from the throat regions.
- Do it for five or nine times of slow inhalation and exhalations. After that, start breathing normally, focusing your mind on your breath only and meditate for fifteen, thirty, or sixty minutes.

Benefits

The main benefits of ujjayi pranayama meditation include curing tonsillitis, breathing problems like asthma, sneezing, etc. It can cure thyroid and parathyroid hormone problems, etc. The best practice of curing all mental issues like anxiety, depression, insomnia, agitation, and wandering of the mind. The best during pregnancy to support pain and normal delivery.

c. Brahmari Pranayama Meditation

Practice

- Hold chin mudra on both hands first and sit for a few breaths, till the mind calms down and breathing becomes normal.
- Now, hold shanmukhi mudra with both hands (closing the ears with the tips of the thumbs, closing the lips with little fingers, partially closing the nostrils with your ring fingers, closing the eyelids with your middle fingers, and place your index fingers on eyebrows).
- Next, inhale slowly, deeply, and then while exhaling partially, close the nostrils and chant M-kara or female bee sound (brahmari).
- Repeat the inhalation flow by chanting M-kara for five times.
- After that release, hold chin mudra on both hands and keep the hands at the knees.

- Start mentally observing the vibrations within, breathe at the nostrils, and meditate for fifteen, thirty, or sixty minutes. Close the session with an ending prayer.

Benefits

- It relieves stress and cerebral tension.
- It reduces anger, anxiety, depression, insomnia, and high blood pressure.
- The best pranayama meditation practice for all psychosomatic problems.
- Spiritual benefits include the deepening of three-dimensional awareness and induce deep meditativeness.

3. Shoonya Meditation (Silent Meditation)

Shoonya meditation is usually practiced after a set of physical postures and breathing exercises, and involves sitting with eyes closed and engaging in a process of conscious nondoing that distinctly creates a distance between one's self and one's body and mind.

Shoonya meditation can be considered as a form of open-awareness practice with self-transcending occurring through a nondoing aspect or conceived as a focused practice in that the explicit focus is on "nondoing"—as soon as one notices mental content arising in awareness, the injunction is to attempt to reinstate a "nondoing"/ nothingness experience and to use a mantra if necessary to do so. Alternatively, within the Isha yoga tradition, this practice is spoken of as a self-transcending practice and maybe in line with the proposed self-transcending style of practice.

Practice

- Take a shower/bath before starting the practice and wear white clothes.

- Apply sandal paste as bindi in between the eyebrows on your forehead.
- Sit on sukhasana or any suitable meditative posture. First, focus on your body parts from down to top as an observer and try to relax all your muscles from toe to head till you feel reasonably comfortable.
- Close your eyes and mouth very softly, concentrate minutely on your forehead and just see the thought if any, and observe until you feel that there is no visible thought.
- Chant OM mantra in the mind silently twenty times to correct your flow of breathing.
- Focus at the tip of your nostril and simply observe your breathing intently without any effort. Do not try anything and just see the pattern. Do not move your body. There should not be any noise or other disturbance that may divert your attention.

You need to start the meditation for thirty minutes in the first week and then for one hour.

Benefits

- Increases concentration and focus
- Gives the feeling of complete relaxation and gentleness
- Mental clarity and alertness
- Reduces body consciousness
- Increases awareness and expand self-consciousness

4. Japa Meditation

Japa means recitation of any bija mantra (means seed or basic mantra, which is OM), mantra, name of God, name of guru, etc. Japa usually starts by fixing a final number before starting. One can choose the number, like 9 times, 21, 27, 54, 108, or 1008. These are important specific numbers. If you miss any number, you have to start again from the beginning. Chanting any mantra for 108 times is considered auspicious and spiritually powerful. For counting, one can use their fingers or japa mala with beads. After chanting for certain numbers, stop chanting and meditate on the vibration or breath, which leads to meditation. This is japa meditation.

Practice

- Sit with eyes closed in any comfortable meditative posture with chin mudra or any other mudra on both hands placed on the laps or at the knees.
- Breathe normally for few times till the breath becomes normal and relaxed.
- Start chanting any mantra such as OM or OM namah shivaya or gayatri mantra or maha mrityunjaya mantra, etc.
– Beginners should chant orally (vachika).
– Then, after some time, with practice, chant by whispering with lips (upamshu).
– Advanced practitioners chant mentally (manasika) for any fixed number like 9, 27, 54, 108, or 1008 times. Odd numbers are recommended.
- Experienced practitioners will go to ajapa japa state, where recitation happens internally without any effort.
- After completion of the chanting, continue the sitting with eyes closed with normal breathing, with a focus of mind on breathing and vibrations within.
- Meditate this way for fifteen, thirty, or sixty minutes. Close the session with an ending prayer.

Benefits

- Japa meditation gives health to the manomaya kosha (mental body)
- Releases mental stress and gives peace of mind
- Releases emotional stress and gives emotional stability

- Chanting sessions accompanied by musical instruments can increase devotion, elevates the mind and self, and removes fear and insecurity of the mind

5. Trataka Meditation

Trataka is the gazing of a flame for a few seconds and meditates on its inner image for long. Trataka is one of the shat kriya to cleanse the eyes and ocular system and the related brain areas. Tratak meditation is a very powerful meditation to stimulate the ajna chakra (eyebrow chakra), which is known as the third eye. Third-eye vision is very important for spiritual sadhakas for seeing beyond the physical aspects of life.

Trataka (Sanskrit, trāṭak: "look, gaze") is a yogic purification (a shatkarma) and a tantric method of meditation that involves staring at a single point such as a small object, the symbol of OM, black dot, or candle flame. It stimulates the "third eye" (ajna chakra) and promotes various psychic abilities.

Practice

- Place a lighted candle at a one-meter distance with the flame at your eye level.
- Sit in a comfortable meditative posture with the hands on the knees in jnana or chin mudra. Keep the eyes closed and breathe normally till you feel relaxed.
- Look down, open your eyes, start moving the eyes toward the candle, and look at the flame for ten seconds. Do not close or blink eyes, even if the tears roll down.
- After ten seconds, close your eyes with both palms softly without touching the eye balls and watch the flame image in the middle of the eyebrows.
- Continue it till the flame afterimage disappears,
- Then remove the hands and open your eyes.

- Again, slowly look at the tip of the wick of the candle intensely for ten seconds.
- Repeat numbers four, five, and six systematically again.
- Then start looking at the aura of the flame for ten seconds.
- Then close your eyes with your palms without touching the eye balls and observe the afterimage of the flame between the eyebrows till it disappears.
- After that, chant OM for three or seven times with the focus on the vibration of the chanting.
- Slowly bring your hands down on your knees and start meditating for fifteen, thirty, or sixty minutes.
- Close the session with a prayer for peace.

Benefits

- Improves eyesight
- Cures headache (like migraine), mental stress, and tension
- Improves concentration
- Increases mental clarity and alertness
- Stimulation and activation of the third eye (ajna chakra)
- Gain of psychic powers like third-eye vision to perceive things beyond physical

6. Shambhavi Meditation

Shambhavi meditation is practiced by adopting shambhavi maha mudra, which is a mahamudra (maha means 'great', and mudra refers to gesture), mudra practiced with the use of mind. This is the most common practice of meditation and is the most powerful meditation practice to invoke the self within.

Shambhavi mahamudra meditation begins with pranayama (controlled yogic breathing) called sukha pranayama or nadi shuddhi, which is an alternate nostril breathing technique (i.e., slow-paced pranayama) to encourage balance in the mind for six to seven minutes, followed by twenty-one long repetitions of the bija mantra (root syllable) OM chanting.

Practice

- Sit in any comfortable posture with eyes closed.
- Breathe for few times till the breath becomes normal.
- Practice nadi shuddhi or sukha pranayama for seven or nine cycles.
- After that, slowly roll your eyeballs upward, keeping the eyes closed, and start mentally looking at the middle of the eyebrows, at the point of ajna chakra. This is shambhavi maha mudra.
- Then chant OM, slow and long, for twenty-one times.
- After that, start meditating on the ajna chakra by looking mentally at the ajna chakra point for a few minutes. If there's any pain in the eyes, relax the eyeballs by bringing the eyes normally.
- Close the session with an ending prayer.
- Meditate for twenty-one minutes daily.

Benefits

- Increases mental clarity and mental alertness
- Improves concentration
- Reduces body consciousness and increases the self-consciousness
- Deepens the awareness and expands the consciousness
- A powerful technique for achieving the realization of the self

7. Vipassana Meditation

Vipassana is a gentle yet profound method of meditation. It is an observation-based journey for self-exploration that focuses on the deep interconnection between the mind and body, which is realized through disciplined attention to the physical sensations, with the main focus on the sensations of breathing at the nostrils. This is the anapana meditation, which is the awareness of the natural breath coming in and going out.

Vipassanā (pāli) or vipaśyanā (Sanskrit), which literally means "special-seeing" (special (vi) and seeing (passanā)), is a Buddhist term that is often translated as "insight." The *Pali Canon* describes it as one of two qualities of mind that are developed (bhāvanā) in Buddhist meditation, with the other being samatha (equanimity, that is, mind-calming). In short, the idea of a vipassana retreat (often referred to as a "sit") is that you sit all day long and learn to sharpen your awareness of what's going on inside your body at the level of sensations. Observation of breath continuously and the sensations created from the process of breathing are mainly focused in this practice.

In 1969, Satya Narayan Goenka started teaching vipassana in India. Seven years later, in 1976, he opened his first meditation center called Vipassana International Academy, also known as Dhamma Giri, at Igatpuri near Nasik in Maharashtra, India.

Vipassana is an awareness or insight-based meditation. You simply observe the nature of reality as it is. By practicing vipassana, you can understand better about your thoughts and find solutions to all your problems.

Practice

- Sit in a very quiet place. Sit in any comfortable meditative posture with spine erect, with eyes closed and hold chin mudra on both hands.
- Breathe normally and start observing your breath, both inhalation and exhalation, throughout your practice. One has to observe the sensations of breathing at the nostrils.
- Observe all bodily sensations, like itching, strain, pain, etc., that are feeling all over the body, if there is.
- Do not respond to any of the physical sensations or mental activities like thoughts coming and going, irritation, worries, happiness, etc.

- Stay relaxed and at ease and be a witness of all physical and mental activities that are going on from a distance of inner space.
- Sit for fifteen, thirty, or sixty minutes. If possible, sit all day long.
- Conclude the session with a prayer of peace for all.

Benefits

- Develops mental clarity and mental alertness
- Develops equanimity to all life's process and toward all people around
- Gets rid of raga-dvesha (likes and dislikes), which is the root cause of karmic bondage and all problems of physical and mental
- Improves control of the senses and attains the state of prathyahara, which will prepare you for intense meditation
- Progresses in the path of yoga to self-realization

8. Transcendental Meditation

Transcendental meditation (TM) refers to a specific form of silent, mantra meditation, and to the organizations that constitute the transcendental meditation movement. Maharishi Mahesh Yogi created and introduced the TM technique and TM movement in India in mid-1950s.

The history of transcendental meditation (TM) and the transcendental meditation movement originated with Maharishi Mahesh Yogi, founder of the organization, and continues beyond his death (2008).

Transcendental meditation is an advanced meditation technique that involves silently repeating a mantra for fifteen to twenty minutes a day and is commonly done sitting with the eyes closed. The technique is not new in the path of yoga, as "transcend" means going beyond your physical and mental nature and merge your self one with the supreme self.

Practice

- Sit in a comfortable posture on the yoga mat with chin mudra on both hands.
- Keep your eyes closed and breathe normally for a few times till you feel relaxed.
- Then, open your eyes and then close them again. Keep the eyes closed during the twenty-minute practice.
- Repeat any mantra in your mind. OM or OM namah shivaya or any other mantra.
- When you see that you are having a thought, simply return to the mantra. Meditate for twenty minutes.
- After twenty minutes, close the session with a prayer for peace.

Benefits

- Improves sleep quality and cures insomnia
- Improves pain management
- Increases mental clarity and alertness
- Rejuvenates and energization the body and mind
- Increases mental focus and productivity
- Increases self-esteem and high concentration

References

1. https://news.harvard.edu/gazette/story/2011/01/eight-weeks-to-a-better-brain/
2. https://www.ncbi.nlm.nih.gov/pmc/articles/PMC6008507/
3. https://www.nih.gov/news-events/nih-research-matters/sleep-deprivation-increases-alzheimers-protein
4. https://www.ncbi.nlm.nih.gov/pmc/articles/PMC4257134/
5. https://pubmed.ncbi.nlm.nih.gov/29632177/
6. https://www.ncbi.nlm.nih.gov/pmc/articles/PMC6595048/
7. https://www.ncbi.nlm.nih.gov/pmc/articles/PMC3746283/
8. https://pubmed.ncbi.nlm.nih.gov/31622587/
9. https://pubmed.ncbi.nlm.nih.gov/18755259/
10. https://www.researchgate.net/publication/51649581_Anti-Parkinsonian_effects_of_Bacopa_monnieri_Insights_from_transgenic_and_pharmacological_Caenorhabditis_elegans_models_of_Parkinson's_disease
11. https://www.ncbi.nlm.nih.gov/pmc/articles/PMC3548360/
12. https://www.researchgate.net/publication/318041805_Asoka_Herbal_Boon_to_Gynecological_Problems_An_Overview_of_Current_Research
13. https://www.researchgate.net/publication/279574592_Herbal_antitussives_and_expectorants_-_A_review
14. https://www.liebertpub.com/doi/abs/10.1089/acm.2015.0272
15. https://www.ncbi.nlm.nih.gov/pmc/articles/PMC3048237/
16. https://www.ncbi.nlm.nih.gov/pmc/articles/PMC4278133/

17. Approach to Neurological Disorders in Ayurveda by Bishnu Choudhary, North Eastern Hill University. https://www.researchgate.net/publication/335796185_APPROACH_TO_NEUROLOGICAL_DISORDER_IN_AYURVEDA

18. Ashtanga Hridayam, By Vagbhata. Translated to English by Dr. R. Vidyanath. https://archive.org/details/AstangaHrdayam.Eng/

19. Hatha Yoga Pradipika by Swami Swatmarama. https://www.yogavidya.com/Yoga/HathaYogaPradipika.pdf

20. https://www.nhp.gov.in/ayurveda_mty (Indian National Health Portal)

21. www.ncbi.nlm.nih.gov/pmc/articles/ (Indian National Health Portal)

22. https://www.yogajournal.com/

23. https://www.spineuniverse.com

24. https://www.msdmanuals.com

25. Andre Van Lysebeth (1974), Yoga Self-Taught. Vikas Publishing, Delhi, India.

26. Timothy McCall, MD (2007), Yoga as Medicine, Bantam Book. New York, USA.

27. Vithaldas Modi (1985), Nature Cure for Common Diseases, Orient Paperbacks, Delhi, India.

28. Swami Satyananda Saraswati (2009), Asana Pranayama Mudra Bandha. Yoga Publication Trust. 4th Edition. Munger, Bihar, India.

29. M.M. Gore. (2016), Anatomy and Physiology of Yogic Practices. New Age Books, Delhi, India.

30. Dr. Vishwas Mandlik (2000), Yoga Therapy-A Practical Guide for the Twenty-first Century

31. Swami Ramdev (2006), Pranayama (Its Philosophy & Practice). 2nd Edition. Divya Yog Mandir Trust. Kankhal, Uttaranchal, India.

32. Patanjali Yoga Sutra, Commentary by Swami Vivekananda. https://www.pdfdrive.com/the-yoga-sutras-of-patanjali-by-swami-vivekananda-e17534288.html

33. Gunaji, N.V., (1999). The Wonderful Life and Teachings of Sri Sai Baba. Adapted from the Original Marathi Book Sri Sai Satcharitha, By Govind Raghunath Dabholkar alias Hemadpant. English

Translation. Published by Shri Sai Sansthan Trust, Shirdi, Mumbai. p. 1-251.

34. Sri Sri Sri Ganapati Sachchidananda Swamiji. Sri Guru Geetha. https://dattadigambara.com/sri-guru-gita/

35. Brian Dana Ankers (2002). The Hatha Yoga Pradipika. Original Sankrit by Svatmarama. English Translation. YogaVidya.com, P.O. Box Woodstock NY 12498-0569 USA. YogVidya LLC. All Rights Reserved. https://www.yogavidya.com/Yoga/HathaYogaPradipika.pdf

36. https://en.wikipedia.org/wiki/Trataka

37. https://en.wikipedia.org/wiki/S._N._Goenka

38. https://en.wikipedia.org/wiki/Transcendental_Meditation

www.ingramcontent.com/pod-product-compliance
Lightning Source LLC
Chambersburg PA
CBHW020523290526

45786CB00002B/739